PSYCHIATRY DISRUPTED

Psychiatry Disrupted

Theorizing Resistance and Crafting the (R)evolution

Edited by
BONNIE BURSTOW,
BRENDA A. LeFRANÇOIS,
AND SHAINDL DIAMOND

McGill-Queen's University Press
Montreal & Kingston · London · Chicago

© McGill-Queen's University Press 2014

ISBN 978-0-7735-4329-4 (cloth)
ISBN 978-0-7735-4330-0 (cloth)
ISBN 978-0-7735-9030-4 (ePDF)
ISBN 978-0-7735-9031-1 (ePUB)

Legal deposit second quarter 2014
Bibliothèque nationale du Québec

Reprinted 2019

Printed in Canada on acid-free paper that is 100% ancient forest free
(100% post-consumer recycled), processed chlorine free

This book has been published with the help of a grant from the Canadian
Federation for the Humanities and Social Sciences, through the Awards to
Scholarly Publications Program, using funds provided by the Social Sciences
and Humanities Research Council of Canada. Funding has also been received
from the Memorial University of Newfoundland.

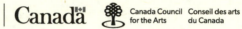

We acknowledge the support of the Canada Council for the Arts.

Nous remercions le Conseil des arts du Canada de son soutien.

Library and Archives Canada Cataloguing in Publication

Psychiatry disrupted: theorizing resistance and crafting the (r)evolution/
edited by Bonnie Burstow, Brenda A. LeFrançois, and Shaindl Diamond.

Includes bibliographical references and index.
Issued in print and electronic formats.
ISBN 978-0-7735-4329-4 (bound). – ISBN 978-0-7735-4330-0 (pbk.). –
ISBN 978-0-7735-9030-4 (ePDF). – ISBN 978-0-7735-9031-1 (ePUB)

1. Antipsychiatry. 2. Psychiatry – Social aspects. 3. Psychiatry – Political
aspects. 4. Psychiatry – Moral and ethical aspects. I. Burstow, Bonnie,
1945–, author, editor of compilation II. LeFrançois, Brenda A., 1968–,
author, editor of compilation III. Diamond, Shaindl, 1980–, author,
editor of compilation

RC454.4.P863 2014   616.89   C2014-900875-9
                                           C2014-900876-7

This book was typeset by Interscript in 10.5/13 Sabon.

For those who inspire us – psychiatric survivors, antipsychiatry activists, and mad activists everywhere.

Contents

Acknowledgments

The editors would like to acknowledge the work of the many people and organizations whose assistance along the way has made this book possible. First and foremost, we would like to acknowledge the efforts of psychiatric survivors and other activists whose sterling work over the years underpins much of the theorizing. We could not have theorized, nor would anyone be writing in this area, if the stories of survivors had not moved us and if their strategic efforts had not tutored us. We likewise acknowledge the various contributing authors whose chapters make this book what it is. Whether it be theorizing trans resistance or the efforts of progressive psychologists, thank you for rising to the occasion and agreeing to be part of the team putting out this ground-breaking book. We thank the kind and expert staff at McGill-Queen's University Press and would particularly like to single out the helpful work of our acquisition editor Jacqueline Mason and editor Kathryn Simpson. We were likewise blessed with exceptional graduate assistants who networked with authors, edited, gathered information as needed, worked long hours so that deadlines could be met – Laura McKinley, Lauren Spring, Griffin Epstein, and the graduate assistant without whose expert knowledge of the Chicago Manual we would have been in dire distress – the multi-talented Mary Jean Hande. We acknowledge the assistance provided by the Ontario Institute in Studies in Education for providing Burstow with four one-year graduate assistantships. This book has been published with the help of a grant from the Federation of the Humanities and Social Sciences, through the Awards to Scholarly Publications

Program, using funds provided by the Social Sciences and Humanities Research Council of Canada, and we would like to thank SSHRC. Publication of this book has been supported by funding from the Memorial University of Newfoundland, whom we additionally thank.

Foreword

PAULA J. CAPLAN

Activism to improve the way we deal with emotional suffering is essential, and the time for it is now. This book's title announces that revolution is needed, given the magnitude of past, current, and – unless we act now and act large – future suffering.

Many of us have spent decades writing and speaking about the harm done by not all but far too many professionals, but far too little has changed. Let me offer a perspective from my experience, and keep in mind as you read that I am only one of a great many who have tried to impel significant improvements and are saddened by the paucity of progress despite massive public education, and by marked increases in the harm caused by some whose job is to help.

I was at American Psychiatric Association headquarters as it prepared an edition of its *Diagnostic and Statistical Manual of Mental Disorders (DSM)* in the mid-1980s, thereby falling through a rabbit hole into the realm of psychiatric diagnosis, where I learned of a myriad of problems that can cascade from the applying of a mental disorder label. The diagnostic system is the *first cause* of everything bad that happens in the mental health system, because labeling is used to justify "treatments" that are often damaging and destructive. If the powers-that-be deem you normal, there's much less they can do to hurt you. I started a petition protesting two proposed DSM categories that would have been especially dangerous to women. The petition ultimately represented more than six million people, but virtually nothing changed (Caplan, 1995). Decades later, I started a change.org petition called "Boycott the DSM: A Human Rights Issue" (http://www.change.org/petitions/boycott-the-dsm-a-human-rights-issue), and nothing changed.

I learned from the inside about the enterprise of creating diagnostic categories when I spent two years on two *DSM-IV* committees, resigning in horror after seeing how starkly *DSM-IV* head Allen Frances and his cronies misused junk science to suit their purposes and ignored, distorted, even lied about good research that conflicted with their aims. I tried using the power of theatre and created videos about harm from diagnosis, created a website and a Facebook page and a blog, organized two Congressional briefings, and called for Congressional hearings, but nothing changed. I have tried in vain for decades to find lawyers who will file lawsuits against the APA and to explore ways to stop the harm caused by the psychiatric diagnoses in the *DSM* and *International Classification of Diseases*.

I organized the filing of nine ethics complaints with the APA's Ethics Committee, describing how complainants had been damaged because of the false advertising of the *DSM* as scientific and helpful and the failure to warn of the harm it often causes. They summarily dismissed the complaints on highly spurious grounds, with no attention to their merits. Despite dismissing the complaints, they could have made restitution and implemented the complainants' many suggestions to prevent future harm, but they did nothing. When four of us went peacefully to APA headquarters simply to request a meeting, someone apparently ordered security guards to eject us from the building. Five of the complainants also filed complaints with the Office of Civil Rights of the United States Department of Health and Human Services, since psychiatric diagnosis is *entirely unregulated* – a fact that ought to be universally known, and that Department is the obvious one that should be providing regulation. At this writing, while we await word of their decision, we are exploring a possibility for complaints to a quite different government entity. After all this and the work of many others, so far, nothing has changed. As Parker warns in this book, massive social change can seem impossible, but, says Parker, it is dangerous in the face of the slow pace of change to ignore the need for radical social changes and escape into the "psy-" realm instead, portraying social problems erroneously as individual, psychological ones.

This book is thus sorely needed and offers a glorious array of forms of activism, some clearly descending from the work of psychologist and feminist Phyllis Chesler. Chesler (1972) in her pioneering *Women and Madness* compellingly exposed and cried out for abolition of many abuses in the so-called mental health system, including but not limited to its prejudices and human rights deprivations. In founding, respectively, MindFreedom International and PsychRights, David Oaks and James Gottstein created vehicles for radical change, MindFreedom through public education and actions like the famous hunger strike (which revealed as unfounded the psychiatric establishment's claim that emotional suffering is caused by chemical imbalances), and PsychRights through filing of courageous lawsuits against Pharma and involuntary commitment.

Many of the chapters reveal that it is about far more than psychiatry specifically. Some therapists – pastoral counsellors, social workers, psychologists, marriage and family therapists, nurses, or psychiatrists – have been compassionate and helpful to those who suffer, and some have done so without pathologizing them. But too many in each category have caused far too much harm.

As Burstow and LeFrançois write in their chapter, the harm is disproportionately done to women – as well as, as Diamond shows in her chapter, to old, racialized, trans, and/or poor people and children but also even to white, heterosexual, wealthy men. The harm comes in a wide array of forms, including but not limited to skyrocketing self-doubt, shame, loss of custody of one's children, loss of employment, and loss of the right to make decisions about one's medical and legal affairs. In this book we see other kinds of harm, perhaps all due to what Withers astutely describes as the relative powerlessness that can result from being called mentally ill. Minkowitz displays her incisive thinking and dynamic leadership in the struggle for international recognition of human rights violations of people regarded as mentally ill, writing that "disability is treated as a disqualification for the exercise of fundamental human rights and freedoms" and showing where mistreatment constitutes torture. Chapman, in a courageously confessional chapter, describes having perpetrated violence against disabled Aboriginal children because of being wrongly taught by others that "our violence was only ever a response to [the children's] violence." Finkler shows how, because of having been labeled "mentally ill," a group of people sharing a residence was subjected to oppressive laws not applied to others. Diamond and Kirby address the damage caused by the pathologizing of people for being transgendered or transsexual, and they note the disturbing phenomenon, due to the psychiatrizing of society, that some people who have suffered because of being considered abnormal actually *seek* psychiatric labels as "evidence" that they have been so mistreated as to become mentally ill. This sad pattern parallels the knee-jerk diagnosing of those who have been to war, raped, or injured in automobile accidents or lived through natural disasters as mentally ill with "Post-traumatic Stress Disorder," which is officially listed as a mental disorder. We ought to offer suffering people help and support without insisting that they agree to be called mentally disordered.

To read this book is to learn about a host of avenues for activism. Mills relates how two people pathologized in the system found ways to resist individually. Adam offers examples of nurses whose radical thinking has led to sorely needed critiques of mental health practices (great models for others who wish to become activists), as well as analysis of why so few nurses have done such work. Beresford and Menzies urge academics to recognize the importance of the knowledge and perspectives of service users/survivors in creating research aimed at bringing about radical change, and McKeown, Cresswell, and Spandler illustrate and call for more "reciprocal democratic" alliances between mental health workers and psychiatric survivors. Finkler describes the inspiring way that mental health survivors living together pronounced themselves a family in order to challenge land-use laws, and Diamond and Kirby show the need for service providers to follow the lead of some in Canada who refuse to call being transgendered or transsexual a mental illness. Barnes and Schellenberg inspire us to turn to alternative approaches to reducing human suffering, showing the importance of speaking and thinking in terms of "emotional pain" rather than "psychiatric disorder" and using art events to treat such pain with respect rather than shaming, to promote healing through the arts by finding or creating meaning, to inspire others to do the same, and to educate the public about the varieties of human suffering. Minkowitz's call to recognize the Convention on the Rights of Persons with Disabilities and apply these rights to those diagnosed as mentally ill reveals a crucial and international arena in which activists can join the struggle. Providing important context for all activism, Burstow cautions that in planning actions, we must avoid legitimizing the currently harmful system and widening its net, and she suggests numerous effective forms of activism, including many through the legal system.

With the publication of this treasure trove of a book offering many avenues for activism, no one can claim that they want to act but don't know what to do. Each of us has a moral responsibility to choose a route to stopping the harm.

Preface

There is a certainty about Burstow, LeFrançois, and Diamond that could only have come from Canada. Psychiatry in whatever guise is the enemy of common sense, reasonableness, empathy, even imagination. It is breathtaking. It's like the old days. Like Szasz, when psychiatry was understood as a means of social control, a kind of voodoo, an invasion of state power upon the individual will struggling with life, with death and debt and unemployment, with the indifference of humanity. Now another element was added.

The evidence of the state that one was unbalanced, crazy, inappropriate, "out of control," insane, incompetent; a danger to one's self or others, and that was that. Then another will imposed, substituted judgment. It no longer matters what you think. You were a "nut case," barely human; every notion you had was only proof that you were "loco."

As for their big new stuff, electroshock? I recognized this was torture when I was only eighteen years old and working at a summer job at St Peter's Asylum in Southern Minnesota. I refused to participate, whereupon I was transferred to night duty in the geriatric ward, waking up old women to a day of nothingness. We ran out of clothes half way through dressing them. Nothing so concentrates the mind to one's humiliation as going naked all day long. Similar situations pertain in private homes even today.

The cruelty of psychiatry has not changed. It has overwhelmed us: where Big Pharma sponsors everything, every conference, every psychiatric journal, and corrupts law enforcement, even immigration.

In hospitals there is still the Thorazine Thirst, caffeine is no longer served on the ward; you can lie in your own waste all day, hoping a nurse will stop by and clean you up, you will eat what they want you to. Management is unafraid to torment you. Forget freedom of movement. There is solitary confinement and bondage, additional punishments and preventions. Don't even dream of sexuality or alcohol, listening to music, or enjoying nature. Life has increasingly less to offer, the life of a prisoner without the thrill of wrongdoing. A confusion of noise, always someone is screaming, yelling, protesting; it never stops. The guards go home to quiet. The prisoners never do.

Elsewhere in the system there is the torment of trans people, their fear of psychiatry, in the definition of personhood, in the permission to surgery, bars often insuperable to their youth and poverty. Then there is the oppression described by Tina Markowitz, as a form of torture as the United Nations saw the Disability Convention work its way through the nations of the world, emerging at last, triumphant. A model for all States to follow, yet few do. Especially now in the face of worldwide recession with migration problems besetting us, warring factions of religion, the rights of women and racialized others so jeopardized. How will we proceed?

Psychiatrists are rarely sued, though they should be. They will respond with a prescription pad, another pill, another bit of medicine to swallow, another part of the self, condemned by them. No matter how proud you are, they'll put you down, they'll settle your case, they will humiliate and patronize you.

I have observed this through three generations of women in my own family – and the friends around me. Psychiatry is very hard on women. There is a double standard, a set of patriarchal practices. They are always at the ready to prescribe, usually having no notion of the effects of the prescription; they will still prescribe it confidently. *Physician do no harm* has no meaning for them. None.

It takes a brave voice to contradict this, to argue the opposite. How necessary this clear call for justice, for common sense against superstition and folly, the casual cruelty of everyday behavior. Intent even in understanding the workings of the mind and finding that useful and admirable. Instead of merely condemning, asking why and how and actually wanting to know.

Barnes and Schellenberg's emphasis upon the arts is especially important. The way the arts give an opportunity to bridge the gap between the public and emotional suffering, nominating it as something everyone experiences. An image in a painting, a gesture in a dance, an evocation of loneliness or despair or joyfulness. The gesture itself, devoid of all syntax, held for a moment so that any observer can give its own meaning.

What is most important about the contributors to this volume is their readiness to experiment, to emphasize, to inquire, to drop the entire pretense to science and sanity, to be honest, to look chicanery in its face and to call quackery by its name. To tell the experience of the people they report on truthfully and in experiential detail. Not as miracle workers with some formula to sell, some special point of view, some theory. They turn much of the accepted wisdom about the human mind on its head, which is as it should be. So much of it is nonsense, propaganda for a guild, even for corporate entities.

This is a landmark book, testimony to honourable research and humane understanding. What is remarkable, almost miraculous, is the sensibility that produced it, that steadfastness in its editors and contributors, that precision, that argument. That these three academics – Burstow, LeFrançois and Diamond – could come up with something this amazing, groundbreaking – this is a book that will be talked about for a long time.

PSYCHIATRY DISRUPTED

1

Impassioned Praxis:
An Introduction to
Theorizing Resistance to Psychiatry

BONNIE BURSTOW AND
BRENDA A. LeFRANÇOIS

Psychiatry is not about benevolence, care, or help. While psychiatric apologists such as Edward Shorter (1997) have long positioned psychiatry as the liberators of the mad, in actuality psychiatry imprisons and oppresses people labeled "mad" in astronomical numbers. At no time in earlier eras was the number caught within the auspices of the mad professions anywhere near the number today. While psychiatry supporters make reference to the terror of Bedlam[1] – currently still in operation, and the hospital in medieval and Renaissance England synonymous with "booby hatch" and memorialized in Shakespeare's plays (see for example, poor Tom in *King Lear*) – the reality is that at any given time during this period only twenty or thirty people were actually held there; and as Porter (2002) makes clear, most people thought of as mad were allowed to rove the countryside without incarceration and without drugs. Such people were certainly often ill-treated – we are in no way depicting these earlier times as good – but without the relentless infringement that characterizes psychiatric practice today.

The history of psychiatry is the history of a profession that ruthlessly drove out all of its competitors – the women healers, the astrologers, ultimately even the psychoanalysts – and completely medicalized any and all conceptualizations of madness, developing both a "mental illness" construct and a world-wide crisis of iatrogenically created drug addicts. In the epistemological violence of diagnosis, in the chemical violence of drugs that place one's very brain into a strait jacket, psychiatry attacks women. By the same token, it attacks seniors. It attacks racialized people. It attacks trans populations. It attacks children. It attacks poor people. However, what is most pernicious about this institution is that it attacks not only these otherwise oppressed groups, it attacks everyone – all this in the name of help. One need only look at the multiplication of diagnoses in the progressive versions of the *Diagnostic and Statistical Manual* (DSM), to realize that this profession is intent on having more and more people under its auspices. This is an institution that is ultimately about pathologizing and "treating" everyday life.

We stand in a long and proud tradition of resistance. It may be argued that resistance to psychiatry is as old as psychiatry itself, albeit it is not until the nineteenth century that we find clear records of such resistance. In the nineteenth century, American psychiatric prisoner Elizabeth Packard brought a writ of habeas corpus against her husband who attempted to reinstitutionalize her; and, simultaneously, Hersilie Rouy, a psychiatrized woman in France and Mary Huestis Pengilly, a psychiatrized woman in Canada were engaged in similar activism (St-Amand and LeBlanc 2013). However we date it, there has long been not only resistance but organized resistance to this institution. Inmates have demonstrated against it, scholars have written about it. Feminized and racialized people have objected to the targeting of their communities. Historians such as Foucault, moreover, have rigorously sought out and surfaced subjugated knowledges.

At times – and necessarily so – this resistance is tied intimately to identity politics. This has been enormously important and, indeed, the ongoing theorizing and resistance to psychiatry by women in particular has contributed substantially to the unmasking of psychiatry as an untenable, patriarchal, and otherwise oppressive institution. As such, identity politics has an absolutely essential role to play. In no way should that reality ever be questioned. As with all identity politics, however, identity politics in this area can at times tip into being exclusionary – and it is this that we question. The need to keep "other" theorists with "other" identities (or those who refuse to identify) at bay may be most keenly felt by people who openly identify as psychiatric survivors, mad, or "service users." People who identify as such often do not want sane-identified people theorizing or engaging in activism on their behalf. This is understandable given the history of harm, domination, and co-optation by seemingly like-minded radical therapists and academics who have benefitted from inequitable alliances with psychiatrized people over the past half century. The marginalization, by seemingly radical therapists, of psychiatric survivors in the U S A that led to the creation of their psychiatric survivor movement is a clear example of such unconscionable domination. Indeed, there are times in every movement, and there are times in the lives of oppressed people, where it becomes important to keep people who do not share that oppressed identity at bay. Nonetheless, in the long run such divisions do not serve us, do not contribute to the task at hand. Neither is it tenable to artificially create dichotomies and divisions between activists and academics, between the openly psychiatrized and those who may refuse classification of their experiences or those who have escaped psychiatrization. The point is, given that we are all at risk of psychiatrization, we cannot afford to exclude the work and theorizing of anyone engaging in radical and activist scholarship, if we are to succeed. We indeed want to underscore how critical the psychiatric survivor voice is in engaging in a psychiatric survivor analysis (Finkler, 2013). However, identity politics alone will not win this fight – any more than the fight against classism would be won if we understood socialism as something that should only be theorized by and fought for by low-wage earners. While honouring the enormous importance of madness-related identity politics, accordingly, we theorize resistance against psychiatry as we would any other (r)evolution: something that demands the attention of all who are critical and where everyone has a role to play.

We use, and are grateful for, the body of work that has been created to date in this regard. Critical, radical, and mad activist scholars from all disciplines and walks of life have been creating such ammunition precisely by exposing the violence of psychiatry – by showing it as medically unfounded (thank you Thomas Szasz, Peter Breggin, Robert Whitaker, and Sami Timimi); by demonstrating the blatant sexism (thank you Phyllis Chesler, Kate Millett, Jane Ussher, Paula Caplan, Jean Baker-Miller, and Dorothy Smith); by unearthing the racism and indeed the colonialism (thank you Frantz Fanon); by demonstrating the enormous harm done to individual lives (thank you Erving Goffman, David Brandon, Geoffrey Reaume, Don Weitz, and Irit Shimrat); by critiquing the D S M (thank you Stuart Kirk and Herb Kutchins); by unmasking sanism (thank you Michael Perlin,

E.L. Finkler, Jennifer Poole, and Erick Fabris); and by linking it to the larger neoliberal machine and biopower relations (thank you Michel Foucault, Nikolas Rose, Peter Beresford, and Joanna Moncrieff).

What has been created to date is of immeasurable value. What we have not as yet created, though, is a body of literature that theorizes precisely how to resist psychiatry. Knowing your adversary is good but not good enough: you must also know how to disempower that adversary – hence our decision to create this volume.

The title of this book, *Psychiatry Disrupted: Theorizing Resistance and Crafting the (R)evolution*, clearly announces the intent, the content, the mission of this book. It is precisely about creating and theorizing resistance to psychiatry, moreover, creating and theorizing resistance that is organized, that is scholarly, that has the force of a revolution. The contributors in this book go beyond theorizing what is wrong with psychiatry to theorize how we might stop it. In the process, we draw on feminism; on the use of the arts; on Marxism; on anarchism; on anti-colonialism; on anti-racism; on disability studies; on mad studies; on anti-psychiatry; on critical psychiatry; on legal theory; on critical psychology; on trans theories; on prison abolitionist principles; on progressive nursing praxis; and on trade unionism.

The diversity evident in the above list is purposeful and necessary. One dimension of that diversity arises out of the geopolitical. What is significant in this regard is that the individual movements that form part of this global movement have developed differently in different geopolitical and cultural spaces and as a result may at times seem to clash with each other. We have neither standardized the theory nor the language of our contributors but instead stand by the importance of allowing the differences to co-exist. Some differences are in appearance only; for example, in the British context, the term "service user" may often be used to refer to politicized survivors of the psychiatric system whereas in Canada the same term "service user" would tend to indicate an uncritical and pro-psychiatry position. In other cases, the difference is as big as it looks and we are pleased, in this respect, that there is more than one position represented in this book. For example, Minkowitz takes a social model of disability lens, while other writers take a critical disability lens, and Withers takes a radical disability lens. In another example, Cresswell, McKeown, and Spandler essentially take a reformist lens whereas Burstow takes an unmitigated anti-psychiatry lens, which permits only very specific kinds of reforms. As the editors of this book, we ask you to consider all of these varied positions because all constitute important contributions to the (r)evolution. Similar to Karl Marx, who neither created nor advocated for a divisive dichotomy between revolutionary and evolutionary Marxisms but instead acknowledged the crucial role of both in creating a class revolution, we understand that crafting the (r)evolution vis-à-vis psychiatry requires a variety of thoughts and actions, best devised as deeply considered and impassioned praxis. At the same time, inclusion in this book does not mean that we as editors agree with all of the positions taken. Nor are we taking an "anything goes" stance. Instead we suggest that some reformist positions are consistent with the ultimate revolution, while others reinstate or reproduce psychiatry. The positions most critical to this struggle are those that are not simply about tinkering but are based in a fundamental critique of psychiatry.

THEMES

The overriding themes of this book include: patriarchy, racism, colonialism, classism, sexism, cis-genderism, ableism – and the way these intersect with sanism – as well as such themes as rule by bureaucracy, medicalization, and pathologization. What are likewise interwoven throughout this book are the following subthemes specifically related to resistance: macro strategies, co-optation, coalition building, policy, and the use of narrative.

Macro strategies are approached differently by our various contributors. Many draw on social movement theory and practice to make concrete suggestions for strategizing. For example, influenced by left-wing anarchism and Quaker praxis, Burstow systematically draws on the early principles of prison abolitionists to articulate an attrition model that can guide anti-psychiatry practice. Specifically, she comes up with three "defining questions" to ask regarding any activism being considered. She demonstrates in turn how these questions can be used in determining which actions of allies to actively support. By contrast, Parker; Menzies and Beresford; and McKeown, Cresswell, and Spandler all draw on critical psychiatry, Marxist analysis, labour resistance, critical psychology, and anti-liberalism to explore such vital issues as coalition building within the labour movement, and the bringing together of academics and psychiatric survivors. Theorizing in a different vein, Minkowitz and Finkler both use legislation to undermine local policy and current practices, all from a structural vantage point; Finkler draws on land use and housing policies and Minkowitz draws on international disability rights legislation. Rather than focusing wholly on the macro level, Mills, in making linkages with the macro-narratives and strategies of colonized and racialized people, theorizes the everyday covert micro strategies that psychiatrized people may use when it is not safe to use more overt strategies.

Coalition building is a particularly central theme. Indeed, the one thing that all contributors are clear about is that coalitions are necessary and have to be improved. Specific types of coalition proposals that weave in and out of the chapters are coalitions between such groups as the disability movement and the various movements that combat psychiatry (Withers); between the mad movement and the anti-psychiatry movement (Burstow); between the organized labour movement, critical psychiatry, and psychiatric survivor movements (McKeown, Cresswell, and Spandler); between the feminist movement and the various movements that combat psychiatry (Burstow and Diamond); and between trans movements and the anti-psychiatry movement (Kirby). While all see coalition as vital, as people who have been in the trenches, no one sees it as easy. Kirby, Burstow, Diamond, and Withers all caution readers about the importance of coalitions that do not sabotage each other, that do not undermine any of the groups vulnerable to psychiatry or any of the movements with which the psychiatric survivor movement, mad movement, or the anti-psychiatry movement overlap. Diamond calls for sensitive coalition building between all constituencies that are critical of psychiatry, while unearthing problems that are created when constituencies limit themselves to protecting their own group.

Co-optation more generally is a serious concern of many of the authors in this book. A number of writers reference, as an example, the co-optation of the gay liberation movement in the seventies (Kirby, Diamond, Burstow). Others also speak of the co-optation of the feminist movement (Diamond). Burstow, additionally, draws attention to the fact that in trying to procure "services" in areas in which there are few services, co-optation frequently happens. Adams explores the inherent and "natural" co-optation of nurses, which happens by virtue of their being theorized and situated as the "handmaidens" of doctors. Courageously sharing his own narrative, Chapman demonstrates the pull to co-optation that occurs when people work within the psychiatric establishment and the concomitant need to scrupulously examine one's rationalizations.

Contributors dealing with professional and academic strategies approach the issues quite differently. Chapman attempts to insert resistance to dominant practice into the social work classroom, demonstrating how personal narrative and ethics can be used to challenge violent, demeaning, and unreflexive practices. Focusing on nursing, and hoping to inspire other nurses, Adam points to individual nurses as examples of the types of resistance that is possible. Parker's overall approach is to bring academic and survivor critiques to bear on the professional practices of the psy-disciplines, whereas Schellenburg and Barnes bring survivors and professionals together through art in order to interrupt dominant psychiatric understandings and practices. Finally, Menzies and Beresford discuss what academics do to push resistance within the halls of academia while detailing some of the obstacles and opportunities therein.

Another theme that weaves through various chapters is engagement with policy. Finkler uses official policy to sabotage policy through an incorporation of a psychiatric survivor analysis. Minkowitz explores the evolution of international covenants and instruments as they theorize disability and disability rights, with particular emphasis on the Convention on the Rights of Persons with Disabilities and the Report of the Special Rapporteur on Torture; and she suggests that these can be used to challenge current mental health legislation. Kirby problematizes the inclusion – and indeed the domination – of psychiatry in policies around trans medical services.

A final dynamic that plays out in a number of the chapters is the use of narrative. Situating herself within the macro narrative of colonialism, Mills suggests that survivors' resistance may be theorized as anti-colonial resistance – and she delves into how psychiatric survivors can and do resist on a daily basis. By contrast, Barnes and Schellenburg, Withers, and Chapman all use their own personal narratives to make visible how co-optation happens and/or how social movements undermine each other. Withers, for example, uses personal narrative to make visible how the knowledges of those with lived disability are undermined. Barnes and Schellenburg used the visual narrative of one survivor's story to show how the paths taken in the face of deep personal problems are complicated by the horror and complexities of psychiatric violence.

ABSENCES

We have been discussing to date what you *will find* in this book – what is strongly and wonderfully present. At the same time, what is as important as what is present is *what is absent*. One cannot edit a book of this nature without being haunted by and calling attention to the absences – what does not exist that inevitably drifts in and out of what is so clearly present (Sartre 1943). No absence – and we would like to particularly emphasize this – is quite so stark and commonplace as the absence of older people and what might be thought of as a senior's perspective. This absence is particularly worrisome when you consider this alarming reality: there is no constituency so subject to psychiatry as older people. Walk through any nursing hospital and you will be hard pressed to find any senior there who is not on psychiatric drugs. Correspondingly, the vast majority of our seniors, by the time they are eighty, are on psychiatric drugs. What adds to this horror is that they are typically and routinely excluded in almost all theorizing about psychiatry.

We have an analysis of how this comes to be. Anyone who suddenly becomes psychiatrized in the later years is almost inevitably engulfed by the system. Accordingly, they are not visible to other survivors and their allies and play little or no role in the movement. Indeed, elderly survivors who are in the movement are typically people who were psychiatrized in their younger years and it is this that they theorize. While the resulting "absence" in theorizing is understandable, we invite everyone – including ourselves – to do better. It is critical that these voices be heard, and that the situation of elderly psychiatric survivors substantially influences our practice. As Diamond points out, we will all be old one day, which makes us all current or eventual targets of psychiatry. Just as all people who are not currently disabled are simply temporarily able-bodied, all people who have escaped psychiatrization have done so only temporarily.

A further absence is theorizing resistance based on the perspectives of children. Although Chapman discusses psychiatrized children, his narrative remains the perspective of an adult. Regretfully, this absence here reproduces and is representative of the general absence of children's theorizing, children's voices, and even children's active presence within critiques of psychiatry. With the one notable exception of Michener's (1998) book, written at the age of sixteen, that provides a long and detailed narrative of her lived experience at the hands of psychiatric and adult violence, children's writings are neither considered nor sought within activist scholarship that is critical of psychiatry. Although some members of the movements against psychiatry have been psychiatrized as children, and indeed some theorize about this, and narrate their stories, these experiences are nonetheless set in a different time, space, and political culture than what current children live in. As such, these accounts, and the theorizing based on them, are necessarily historical accounts of childhoods past rather than depicting the experiences of current children.

Children are being massively over-drugged as a result of the complex relationships between pharmaceutical companies vested capitalist interests and child psychiatry's subsequently entwined influence over parents, carers, and other professionals working with children (such as within social work, nursing, and education). This influence is made possible by psychiatry's emotive and paternalistically authoritarian posturing of "knowing" what is in the *best interest of the child*. As such, children's standpoints in relation to their lived experience of psychiatric violence remains muted. For the most part, children are excluded from involvement in all of the activist movements against psychiatry. In part this is the direct result of systemic design relating to the adult-centric definition, form, practice, and leadership of these movements,[2] which ultimately are distinct from and exclude children's ways of knowing, children's ways of being, children's ways of relaying information, children's ways of interchanging with each other, and children's ways of organizing collectively. This adultism within the various movements against psychiatry serves to reproduce child psychiatry's reliance on conceptualizing children as incompetent actors, as incapable of producing knowledge, and as unable to function within, and as, a collective. Yet, most children are more than able to demonstrate an activist stance against their oppressors.

Although there are many examples worldwide of children's collective organizing, such as within activists organizations run for and by children in state care and disabled children, psychiatrized children have neither organized themselves in similar ways nor have they played any central part within these related communities. Coalition building – within the children's rights movement, between disabled children's organizations or children in care organizations – with psychiatrized children has not materialized. This has not happened despite the common issues of living in a disabling world and despite the overwhelmingly large number of children in care who have been traumatized by abuse and other forms of adultist violence, which is then reframed as these children suffering from "mental illness." We question whether these exclusions result from sanist attitudes that are perpetuated within these other children's movements by children who have escaped psychiatrization. Although sanism stems from adult culture, it permeates and plays out within children's culture, in ways that further marginalize and isolate psychiatrized children.

Yet another absence from this volume is those psychiatrized people who have specifically been held under the criminal code. Significantly, both people who have been found unfit to stand trial and people who have been found guilty but not criminally responsible almost invariably fall under psychiatric rule. Typically, their psychiatric incarceration continues far longer than most people's and certainly longer than a jail sentence. They are held involuntarily until they are proven to be "not dangerous to society" – and we all know we cannot disprove a negative. That is, dangerousness may be proven by reference to an overt action that is deemed dangerous, whereas proving that one is not dangerous can only be made through reference to the absence of an action, an absence that can never be said or proven to exist indefinitely. This is its own horror and its own trap and resistance to it needs to be theorized.

Equally important, there is also an absence in this volume of the voices of racialized people. Significantly, while some of the authors are indeed people of colour, their chapters are not written specifically from the perspective of racialization. Correspondingly, while there are some very good critiques of racism and the implications of racism (see, for example, both Chapman and Mills) none of the authors identify in this book as members of communities targeted by racism. Given the widespread psychiatric targeting of racialized people, for example the psychiatric attribution of schizophrenia to black people (Metzl, 2011), once again we need to do better. Other racialized voices that we do not hear in this book are Indigenous people, Jews, and members of various other diasporas. Given the (often intergenerational) trauma associated with lived experiences of colonization, the Holocaust, as well as occupation and civil wars, Indigenous people, Jews, as well as refugees, asylum seekers, and people living under occupation, all remain targets for psychiatric oppression – in particular by psychiatry's tactic of individualizing and reframing the distress resulting from state-related violence as biogenetic and bio-chemical induced "mental illness." In this way, psychiatry remains the handmaiden of the state in obscuring the impact of state-sanctioned violence, racism, and greed as well as redirecting attention away from those who ultimately should be made accountable for the distress of so many people.

VOICES

A number of voices and perspectives are loud and clear in this volume. This being an academic book, first and foremost we hear from scholars. Moreover, we hear from scholars of a variety of stripes – sociologists, adult educators, historians, disability theorists, anticolonial theorists, people who theorize from at once within and against the psy-disciplines. While academics are often and we would suggest erroneously distinguished from psychiatric survivors in activist circles as if a person is either one or the other, we particularly hear from psychiatric survivors, each of whom are academics in their own right. We likewise hear from members of trans communities, feminist communities, from organized labourers, activists, and professionals. Most contributors wear more than one hat, often combining activist with theorist, with psychiatric survivor, and oftentimes with professional. It is precisely through reflecting on such complex identities that a fuller analysis emerges.

WEAVING THEORY

We began by looking at the title of the book. We have come full circle and are back again with the title. In subtitling this book "Theorizing Resistance and Crafting the (R)evolution," our evocation of the image of crafting is intentional and multi-dimensional. For one thing, we are calling attention to the fact that whether resistance takes the form of art or the form of labour or labour demonstrations, all praxis that sets about to change the world is necessarily creative. Also, if it is to succeed, it must be intelligent; the word "crafty" signifies a practical intelligence, something generally attributed to classes, genders, races, and ages hegemonically deemed "inferior." Moreover, the concept of "crafty" connects with contributor China Mills' phrase "sly normality." The word craft is also intimately connected to the concept of witchcraft, a term often used to further dismiss, subjugate, and demonize women working outside of medicine, for example women using natural, herbal, holistic, and/or spiritual healing remedies. In addition, for us the word "craft" connotes cottage industry or community-based work, often produced by poor folk, including poor women, poor racialized people, and poor children. Despite lack of finances or material goods, this crafting by poor people often demonstrates resourcefulness, creating the extraordinary out of simple materials found nearby. So too we acknowledge how activism and radical scholarship has worked to produce alternative knowledges, usually without research funding and certainly without corporate sponsorship, all amidst the dominance and privileged positioning of psychiatric and pharmaceutical discourse. We likewise use the word "craft" to acknowledge the seemingly small and daily efforts by which people resist, and we link this up to the way in which women, girls, and other oppressed groups have typically engaged in resistance.[3] In this regard, we call attention to how women and girls in the global north, in the early 1970s (including the two authors of this chapter), talked over their kitchen tables, sometimes while knitting, sometimes while making a tapestry, in some homes, theorizing the patriarchy, while in other homes, plotting their escape from the effects of poverty.

We leave you with one image of a working class woman's resistance that was literally created through and embedded within her craft. Significantly, throughout Charles Dickens' novel *A Tale of Two Cities* one woman can be seen, in scene after scene, knitting – the solitary figure of Madame Thérèse DeFarge. Only toward the end of the novel, do we discover *what* she is actually knitting: a figure in the French revolution, she is knitting the names of which aristocrats are to be beheaded and in which order. While we are in no way calling for such violence, for we all look to this being a revolution of a very different nature, we do connect the concept of the *tricoteuse* with the crafting of the revolution against psychiatry.

In this spirit, as young women, as middle-aged women, and as old women, the editors of this text invite you to read, to enjoy, to ruminate, to disrupt, and most of all, to pick up a thread and add to the tapestry.

NOTES

1 Bedlam is the colloquial term for the Bethlem Royal Hospital which was the first hospital for the "insane" in Europe located in London, England. Historical accounts of Bedlam consist of descriptions of moaning, frenzied, and chained inmates, living in degrading circumstances and filthy conditions, with an inadequate water supply, a frequently backed-up sewage system, and where malnourishment, starvation, and other abuses were the norm. The term "bedlam" has since become synonymous with "chaos," "confusion," "uproar," "irrationality," and even "madness" itself. Still in existence today, albeit in a different location from the original building and in what is characterized as more humane conditions, Bedlam has been operating as a psychiatric hospital for over 600 years.

2 It is also in part related to the lack of access that the movements have to psychiatrized children – who tend to be as socially isolated as elderly psychiatrized people, albeit for different reasons – and the lack of access that these children may have to the adult movements.

3 Also, see Shaikh (2013) for her conceptualization of "crafting" in the context of anti-racist feminist organizations.

2

Becoming Perpetrator:
How I Came to Accept Restraining
and Confining Disabled Aboriginal Children

CHRIS CHAPMAN

INTRODUCTION

Some people may not wish to read this paper. It is an attempt to make sense of my own past perpetration of physical restraints and locked confinement of disabled Aboriginal children. My nightmare scenario of writing this is that it will do harm to people who've been subjected to such violence and read it. If you have been subjected to physical restraints and locked confinement, please know that this is the subject of the following paper, and so you may or may not wish to read ahead. I could never know for you whether or not you should proceed. On the other hand, if, like me, you have perpetrated this kind of violence, then I would encourage you to read it. If you feel defensive or otherwise strongly respond to what I write, I invite you to consider that this may be a response that you can attend to ethically and politically – and that it could possibly be an important response that may not be primarily or only about what I've written. Of course I could never know this for you either.

Hannah Arendt wrote: "What I propose ... is nothing more than to think what we are doing" (1998, 5), which I think fed her subsequent suggestion that a more rigorous understanding of Adolf Eichmann's account of his thinking about what he was doing would have been politically useful for us all. In this paper, I take her analysis of Eichmann's accounts and use it as a starting point to explore resonances with how I thought about what I was doing in the past as a residential counsellor. I then briefly connect this to my work today as a social work instructor and some pedagogical considerations that guide me in that context.

Over ten years ago now, I worked as a residential counsellor in a treatment centre. Elsewhere I've critically explored this work on a more systemic and theoretical level (Chapman 2012), but I've been hesitant to explore my own use of violence directly, in physically restraining children as young as eight and locking them up. I continue to struggle with how I was able to do that. I am not suggesting that I, or other residential counsellors, can be equated with Eichmann, in that this would surely do an injustice to many people in various ways. One of the perhaps less obvious ways it would do so is by taking away from the particularity of the ways that real people navigate real contexts, particularly when any one of us does real harm to any other.[1] I approach Eichmann's accounts, then, as particularly embodied and contextualized narratives of personal ethical navigation – as I understand Arendt to have done. I believe that we all navigate our lives in ways that are available to us, in part due to the structural contexts in which we find ourselves and the stories we tell about ourselves and the world. I believe this is a way to fruitfully approach how anyone lives in this world and does things, whether it's you, or I, or Eichmann. Of course every person's ethical navigations have particular and contingent effects on others, and few people's lives have as devastating consequences on so many other lives as did Eichmann's. Without minimizing the real consequences of people's actions, there's something valuable in carefully attending to the "hows" of ethical navigation – amongst those who do it very carefully, those who do it with devastating consequences, and – like most of us, probably – those who do it carefully sometimes and in certain contexts, and who also sometimes do it with harmful consequences. This kind of analysis is distinct from an approach that imagines that violence and atrocities are always committed by people entirely unlike the rest of us – a view that, I would suggest, implicitly justifies psychiatric and penal abuse and incarceration, as well as war. As an alternative, I'm inviting curiosity about how someone *becomes* an administrator of genocide, how someone else becomes a restrainer and confiner of disabled Aboriginal children, and how we two very different people – and the rest of us when we do harm – come to accept hurting and oppressing others as normal or acceptable, and then go on with our lives. What makes this possible? What might make it less likely to happen?

WHY I BELIEVE IT IS IMPORTANT TO TAKE EICHMANN'S ACCOUNT SERIOUSLY

It's easy for us to imagine that Eichmann was simply a monster. And, of course, he was exactly that in terms of what he did. But *how* he became what he became is another question altogether (see Butler 2004; Patel 2009). According to Arendt, this is more complicated than we might assume. She writes, for example:

> Eichmann pleaded: "Not guilty in the sense of the indictment."
> [and so Arendt asked in what sense he thought] he was guilty ...
> First of all, [he claimed,] the indictment for murder was wrong:
> "With the killing of Jews I had nothing to do [he stated]. I never
> killed a Jew, or a non-Jew, for that matter – I never killed any
> human being. I never gave an order to kill either a Jew or a non-
> Jew; I just did not do it" ... Hence he repeated over and over ...
> that he could be accused only of "aiding and abetting" the anni-
> hilation of the Jews, which he declared in Jerusalem to have been
> "one of the greatest crimes in the history of Humanity." (1964, 25)

Elsewhere (Chapman 2010), I explore this dividing line he draws, using Guatemalan human rights activists' distinctions between "material authors" and "intellectual authors" of genocide (Jesús Tecu Osorio, in al Nakba 2008), in relation to other studies of people who have done harm and the lines they draw to secure their own relative innocence (Fellows and Razack 1998; Goodrum, Umberson, and Anderson 2001; Hatzfeld 2005; Heron 2007; Wood 2004). Here, however, it is the second point of his plea, alongside his statement that the annihilation of the Jews was "one of the greatest crimes in the history of Humanity," that interests me. His second point was this: "The indictment implied not only that he had acted on purpose, which he did not deny, but [that he had acted] out of base motives" (Arendt 1964, 25). He was, he claimed, "not guilty in the sense of the indictment" because the indictment assumed – as I think we all tend to do when we hear of others' violence – that his motivation was clearly, simply, and unambiguously *to do harm*, because he was a certain kind of person unlike the rest of us.

In relation to the idea that a given person "is" a certain kind of person, Michael White (2004a) has provided a very compelling account of the distinction between what he calls "the folk psychologies" that have always existed in all places and all times and the relatively recent, putatively scientific, and Eurocentric "professional psychologies." These new ways of understanding humanity have tended to posit that a core self is to be found in each of us and that what a person does can be understood by interrogating things internal to that person's individual psyche, no matter whether a person is born with these internal characteristics or whether they are aquired through socialization. Often we do not 'know' this self, but it is imagined to be there to be found. This orientation of the professional psychologies would have had no ground to flourish without the likewise relatively recent and Eurocentric liberal individualist understandings of personhood. Heron (2007) notes that liberal individualism enables self-narratives that she describes as a "unitary moral self," according to which one is either good or bad, sane or insane, responsible or irresponsible, and so on. And Foucault (1970) gives more detailed analyses of what made these forms of objectification possible, describing certain developments as occurring "at the level of what will soon be called psychology" (224). Further, he writes that these were not politically neutral developments and that, in fact, case notes taken in asylums were central to the development of liberal individualism:

> We cannot say that the individual pre-exists ... the projection of the psyche, or the normalizing agency. On the contrary, it is ... through disciplinary mechanisms that the individual appeared within a political system. The individual was constituted insofar as uninterrupted supervision, continual writing [i.e., of case notes], and potential punishment enframed this subjected body and extracted a psyche from it. It has been possible to distinguish the individual only insofar as the normalizing agency has distributed, excluded, and constantly taken up again this body-psyche ... The sciences of man, considered at any rate as sciences of the individual, are only the effects of this series of procedures. (Foucault 2008, 56)[2]

There is no reason for us to take for granted the truth claims of these particular ways of understanding what humans are, other than habit. And I would like to suggest that a critique of the objectification that is accomplished through liberal individualism and the professional psychologies coincides with the possibility that Arendt's account of Eichmann may be useful for all of us in understanding how a person becomes violent and oppressive, and especially how a person narrates or rationalizes this process. Foucault writes:

> Many factors determine power. Yet rationalization is also constantly working away at it. There are specific forms to such rationalization. The government of [people] by [people] – whether it is power exerted by men over women, or by adults over children, or by one class over another, or by a bureaucracy over a population – involves a certain type of rationality [at the level, we might add, that has come to be called psychology] ... Consequently, those who resist or rebel against a form of power cannot merely be content to denounce violence or criticize an institution ... What has to be questioned is the form of rationality at stake. The criticism of power wielded over the mentally sick or mad cannot be restricted to psychiatric institutions; nor can those questioning the power to punish be content with denouncing prisons as total institutions. The question is: how are such relations of power rationalized? (1994, 324–5)

It is this rationalization of relations of power that seems to interest Arendt most in her careful study of Eichmann's own narratives. Arendt writes of what we most easily assume to be his anti-Semitism, for example: "He 'personally' never had anything whatever against Jews; on the contrary, he had plenty of 'private reasons' for not being a Jew hater. [And then she adds] Alas, nobody believed him" (1964, 26). This "alas" is very significant to Arendt's project. I believe she's concerned that Eichmann is being misrepresented *for the sake of what we can learn from his example* if what he says *is* true (and even if it is only partially true). I'm following her lead in assuming that what he says is at least partly true and in believing that we can all learn from the ways that he accounts for the process of having ethically normalized and rationalized his own perpetration of violence. Narrativizing this violence as "aiding and abetting" rather than murder or genocide surely played some role in such rationalization. But how did he initially become comfortable with "aiding and abetting" what he called "one of the greatest crimes in the history of Humanity?" He says he did not initially experience this as anything like acceptable: "when he was told of the Führer's order for the 'physical extermination of the Jews,' in which he was to play such an important role[, he says that] he himself had 'never thought of ... such a solution through violence,' and he described his reaction [as follows]: 'I now lost everything, all joy in my work, all initiative, all interest; I was, so to speak, blown out'" (Arendt 1964, 31). Of course we all know that this initial response did not last.

HOW THIS RESONATES WITH HOW I CAME
TO NORMALIZE MY OWN USE OF VIOLENCE

First of all, let me say again that I am not equating myself with Eichmann. When I use the term "resonance" to describe a relationship between our respective processes of normalizing and rationalizing violence, this should not be read as a making of equivalencies. I am rather using this term along the lines of what Tamboukou (2003) calls "dissonant harmony" – which is to say a sense of some commonality that is also very much "dissonant" or distinct. I also relate to Jenkins' (2009) description of "parallel, political journeys" by which he refers to the resonance between his position as a therapist and that of the men who perpetrate abuse that he works with: he's suggesting that his own journey to be accountable for the real effects of his actions on the men he works with and their families is "parallel" to or resonant with the journeys of the men he works with to become accountable to their families' experiences of them. He is not suggesting that he is himself a perpetrator of domestic violence, any more than I'm suggesting that I'm "the same as" Adolf Eichmann. I'm rather attending to very particular ways that I can learn from Eichmann's accounts of his own process, allowing myself to "sit with" what I feel is resonance with his accounts, and using this as a starting point for my own reflexive exploration.

I can still remember the specifics of the first two restraints I ever did – and no others in the same kind of detail. I think these two continue to stand out for me because, as Arendt says of Eichmann, my "conscience [initially] functioned in the expected way" even if, relative to the rest of my life, it functioned "within rather odd limits"

(Arendt 1964, 95). Like Eichmann's, this initial, expected, conscientious response did not last.

I'd sought out a social services job out of a sense of political commitment. I believed that working with "disadvantaged" youth was a way to make a difference in the world – along the lines of something like global justice. When I first started the job, I had no training or experience, but I had a lot of ideas and enthusiasm – which were politically, rather than individualistically, oriented. I imagined watching John Wayne movies with the children and collectively critiquing their racism, for example. And I imagined that doing so might be "therapeutic" because of how I came into the job understanding what it meant to be "disadvantaged." But then I took on the training regime of what I needed to learn to do my job (see also Chapman 2012). And so instead of watching cowboy movies critically and asking the children what they thought, I watched things like "Ten Things to Do Instead of Hitting" (Sunburst 1995) uncritically and then told the children what to do. One of the things that *my* training regime entailed, because of who I'd always been, was ongoing concern about my ability to "set limits," "establish boundaries," and generally discipline and control. I had to learn to be "the adult" in the relationship, even though I'd never had an adult *like that* in my life. And one of the major things this entailed was to physically restrain children.

In fact, untrained and inexperienced, I soon found out that I had basically been hired on as "muscle," which seemed like a joke really. I was also to be a "male role model" to the children, which was likewise a bit of a joke to me, but the concern about male physical strength was explicitly stated. Before I was ever expected to take the lead in education groups or counselling, I took the lead in physical restraints. This because I was a man. Alongside sighs of exasperation about there being no Aboriginal staff – and no serious efforts to address this – the centre had a strict policy that half of the full time staff be male. White women who had worked there casually for years were not hired, no Aboriginal people were considered, and they took my effeminate, university-dropout masculinity as the best they could do. I found myself with a job involving pay and responsibility that was unparalleled amongst my peer group at the time.

As I understood it then, I was actually making a difference in the real lives of survivors of family and colonial violence and getting trained and compensated to do so, and so I was very much "elated" about aspects my situation (see Arendt 1964, 53–4, on Eichmann's strategies for achieving elation, which I address below). But I also had to physically restrain children, which was initially incredibly emotionally complicated for me, and was something which nothing in my previous life had prepared me for. I can remember that when I talked with friends and family, the restraints were a major focus of early conversations. I would state my discomfort about what I was doing, but somehow the self-centred story of the perceived ridiculousness of my body having been chosen to do such a thing often won out. This "my body" completely ignored my whiteness, non-disability, adulthood, and maleness and instead focused exclusively on my effeminacy – the fact that it seemed funny to me that a white, male, non-disabled, adult body was considered appropriate to overpower disabled Aboriginal children clearly shows my sense of disconnect from legacies of colonization and eugenic institutionalization (see Chapman 2012). "Can you believe it," I would say, "they hired *me* to do this? Some of those children are bigger than I am and I've never even been in a fight." This was funny to me, because it was so incongruous with anything else I'd ever done or known, but it was also incredibly disturbing to do these things. And, perhaps even more disturbing, somehow I knew that this disturbance was to be psychologically "worked through" and "overcome" rather than politically and ethically attended to.

BECOMING PERPETRATOR AS A PARALLEL, POLITICAL PROCESS TO BECOMING SELF-BLAMING OTHER

Of the Nazis, Arendt writes that, in terms of affect and ethical self-governance, "the problem was how to overcome ... the animal pity by which all normal [people] are affected in the presence of physical suffering. The trick used by Himmler – who apparently was rather strongly afflicted with these instinctive reactions himself – was very simple and probably very effective; it consisted in turning these instincts around, as it were, in directing them toward the self. So that instead of saying: What horrible things I did to people!, the murderers would be able to say: What horrible things I had to watch in the pursuance of my duties, how heavily the task weighed upon my shoulders!" (1964, 106)

At the treatment centre, it was routinely acknowledged that it was disturbing to physically restrain someone. This was spoken about as an "unfortunate" aspect of the job. If only we could play games and have counselling sessions all day, without the violence, without the time-outs even, of course we would all prefer that. But one of the things that came with helping children who were so damaged, as we narrated the encounter between us and them, was restraining and confining. The idea that there could be a world without restraints and locked confinement seemed clearly untrue, as evidenced by the children we worked with (as we framed and perceived them). As a result, some of us had to do the "unfortunate" work involved – narrated not as violence, but as maintaining safety for them and others. It was not that we did not acknowledge that these restraints were traumatic for the children being restrained or for other children witnessing them, but we were the protagonists in the stories we told and believed. Our violence was only ever a response to their violence. The possibility of imagining their individual violence as a response to our structural, epistemic, *and* individual violence – institutional, disablist, adultist,[3] nationalist, colonialist, and racist – was not available to us. And so because they were the initiators of violence, as we understood it, there was nothing *we* could do to prevent it (see Butler 2004). We had nothing to do with their violence until it erupted; and our only role was to keep everyone safe. Even the room where children were locked up, which usually followed a physical restraint, was called a "safe room," which was clearly an act of manipulating perception – but it's hard to locate the *agent* of that manipulation. As staff, I think we all believed it. We *perceived* it. There was no safety without the safe room, we said, "unfortunately."

"Unfortunately." It seems to me that what was once an ethical and political "crisis of conscience" about what we were doing (Arendt 1964, 104) – for me and perhaps for others – somehow gave way to this resigned "unfortunately," as if it were merely misfortune that placed the children upon the path to the treatment centre rather than the effects of real people's concrete decisions and actions (see Ahmed 2004). As if it were sheer misfortune that created the fact that almost all of them were Aboriginal and almost all of us were white. And, "unfortunately," someone had to "care for them" – with all the sense of righteousness and self-sacrifice that this phrase implied. In fact, while I was there, all of the staff went away on a retreat for "secondary post-trauma" – the trauma experienced as a result of exposure to others' trauma. Doing what was clearly "group therapy," but calling it "professional development," the purpose was for us to explore the effects on us of the stories we heard in counselling conversations, rather than the effects on us of restraining children, but nevertheless I can imagine a different "treatment" of our feelings. Relative to the children we worked with, our traumas were much less significant, but they were nonetheless real. And perhaps they could have instead been taken for what Arendt calls "instinctive reactions" to *both* the painful experiences the children told us about *and* the painful experiences we perpetrated. But by psychologizing and thus depoliticizing our emotional and at least potentially ethical and political struggles, we were actively steered away from interrogating our own violence and the trauma *we were causing*. In her paper for the PsychoUT conference, Louise Tam (2010) cited Mitchell-Brody of the Icarus Project, both of them using the following statement to question the pathologization of people who are psychiatrized: "there is much in our world to be angry, anxious, or sad about." I would like to suggest, here, that the "normal" or "instinctual" or at least expected experiences of anger, anxiety, and sadness that staff experienced were psychologized and abnormalized in a "dissonant" but complementary way to the pathologization of the children we worked with and others who are confined in similar closed sites. Taking up Jenkins' (2009) language differently than he uses it, I would like to suggest that this was a "parallel, political journey" – but it was not one of "becoming ethical" in the sense that "ethical" sometimes means "moral." It was, rather, a process of becoming invested in a project of ethical self-governance that would allow us to more comfortably occupy and perpetuate our respective positions in systemic oppression.

I now consider my worry, guilt, and anger about such things as important. The children I worked with were pathologized of course, making our violence seem necessary, but workers' struggles with perpetrating violence were also psychologized and individualized, thereby steering us away from approaching these struggles as political or ethical concerns. When we restrained children, we "debriefed" newer staff afterwards, knowing it was difficult to witness or participate in a restraint, and approaching it as something to address through something like a "talking cure" with a predetermined destination: to accept perpetrating violence as necessary. The word "debrief," in fact, as I understand it, is primarily otherwise used in military contexts to work through having participated in military violence and all that it entails – and when Global North inhabitants come back from working in the Global South. In the latter, we can imagine that if the discomforts of coming back to Canada from Guatemala were approached as "ethical and political" concerns to attend to, then this would result in a more normative fundamental questioning of geopolitical inequalities, starvation, war, and what Heron (2007) calls "colonial continuities."

In the treatment centre, our expected and therefore "normal" discomforts resulting from restraining were differentiated from those of the children we worked with, which served the purpose of implicitly threatening the staff with the identification of "emotionally disturbed" if we were unable to "work through" our initial discomforts. In fact, this was how we as staff made sense of the "conscientious objector" staff person I describe a few pages below: she was "not right" or "not healthy enough" to do the job, or something along those lines. Our discomforts as staff, however unpleasant, could be worked through "normally," meaning without confinement or restraint, proving that we were worthy of our freedom while the children we worked with, who seemed to need these interventions, were exceptionally, individually disturbed.

This divisibility of normal working through of difficulty from experiencing difficulty pathologically also seems to present itself in other instances where violence is rationalized. A few years ago, I presented on a panel with Shaista Patel (2009) and Melissa Abbey Strowger (2009). Patel's paper explored how "terror suspects" were described in popular press sources using discourses of "madness," which both erased the possibility of understanding "terrorists" as politically motivated and evoked a longstanding tradition of incarcerating people who have committed no crime simply because of their "psychological state." Strowger's paper also looked at popular press sources, although her study was of the ways that Americans' anxiety about "the war on terror" was treated in these sources – anxiety that could, at least potentially, be related to questioning the justice of American military action. This anxiety was unlike the "madness" of the "terror suspects" that self-evidently required incarceration. It was rather, according to some of her sources, to be worked through using "relatively normal" practices often used in outpatient care for those not "requiring" confinement, restraint, and so on: if you're feeling anxious about the war, here are some deep breathing exercises you could do, or you might try positive aphorisms. "Parallel" to one another, and certainly "politically," some are psychologized to accept their own implication in war with less anxiety and uncertainty, and others are psychologized so that the rest of us can accept their indefinite detention and torture. This was a "parallel, political" process to what took place at the treatment centre where I worked; both processes created discursive contexts within which people could engage in ethical practices of self-formation (see Mahmood 2005). These ethical practices would, in turn (Foucault 1980b), reify the naturalization of these discourses of rationality and inevitability and, through them, people would constitute themselves as "willing" to do the material acts also necessary for the sustenance of systemic oppression, such as directly perpetrating violence themselves or electing officials who choose war, indefinite detention, and torture.

Furthermore, resonant with our staff retreat to deal with secondary trauma, and also with newspapers advocating deep breathing and affirmations for anxiety about war, Arendt writes the following of what we might call Eichmann's "positive self-talk":

He had not forgotten a single one of the sentences of his that at one time or another had served to give him a "sense of elation." Hence, whenever, during the cross-examination, the judges tried to appeal to his conscience, they were met with "elation," and they were outraged as well as disconcerted when they learned that the accused had at his disposal a different elating cliché for each period of his life and each of his activities. In his mind, there was no contradiction between "I will jump into my grave laughing," appropriate for the end of the war, and "I shall gladly hang myself in public as a warning example for all anti-Semites on this earth," which now, under vastly different circumstances, fulfilled exactly the same function of giving him a lift. (1964, 53–4)[4]

And what held all the violence, care, and rationalization at the treatment centre together as sensible, but which has no secure foundation, is the myth of achieving an enduring state of normalcy, free from emotional discomfort, even in the face of violence and oppression. The children and staff were both disciplined toward this imaginary state, parallel to one another, but distinctly. Following restraints, we "debriefed" new staff to help them feel at peace with perpetrating these forms of violence; and then we "processed" with the child who had just been restrained, requiring them to accept "full respon-sibility" for having individually caused the entire situation (see Jenkins 1990). Any suggestion from a child that staff, other children, or the system played any part whatsoever in their individual choices or actions, would result in another fifteen minutes of locked con-finement, after which we would give them another opportunity to take "full responsibility" – unless some other duty delayed us, which sometimes happened but was never our responsibility either. Their discursively construed and structurally coerced "responsibility" shaped their – and our – ethical and political possibilities of becom-ing who we were becoming. We were all being trained to more fully inhabit our respective positions within systemic oppression, and to feel fully responsible or not at all, accordingly.

THE IMPORTANCE OF ALTERNATIVE ACCOUNTS TO PROCESSES OF ETHICAL SELF-FORMATION

Significantly, we were not aberrational in our normalization of our particular kind of violence. It is normative, at least for those living in our time and place with systemic privilege, to imagine the inevi-tability of the police, the army, psychiatric confinement, prisons, and so on. I struggled initially with *my role* in this place and practice, but it was not until I left the job that I began to imagine a world without such places and practices. "As Eichmann told it, the most potent factor in the soothing of his own conscience was the simple fact that he could see no one, no one at all, who actually was against the Final Solution. He did encounter one exception, however, which he mentioned several times, and which must have made a deep impression on him" (Arendt 1964, 116).

In terms of encounters with exceptions, critiques, and alternatives, a difference between Eichmann and I is that I had direct and some-times very close relationships with every one of the children I ever restrained. The children very clearly told us as staff that what we were doing to them was "contrary to morality"; they "appeal[ed] to our feelings" (Arendt 1964, 131) in deeds and words of a wide vari-ety of forms and intensities. But one of the things that today I find so astounding in thinking back on this is that all of those words and deeds only served to justify what we were doing (see Chapman 2009; Jenkins 1990, 1991). The necessity of our "Nonviolent Crisis Intervention"[5] was proven by their violence[6] (see also Butler 2004).

Our control of them, and our need for control of them, was rendered completely natural and not the least noteworthy or up for consideration. And the same was true for our violence. This is connected to legacies of disablement, colonization, classism, and adultism. Due to these interlocking forces, the children in the treatment centre could not effectively call our actions into question, no matter how they tried. Even when they questioned our violence and control in calm, articulate, curious ways, or through tears, *even then* we as staff were entirely sure about the morality of what we were doing – or at least its inevitability. This was just how things were, and the only people who could change that were the children: if they were never violent again, we would never be violent – simple.

Unlike Eichmann's solitary exception, I also had access to several critiques from the margins of the staff team. These shook up my certainties more than the children's protests, but it wasn't until I left the job that my uncertainties really flourished. At one point, I visited a former co-worker who had moved away. She had been "night staff," which meant that, according to local beliefs in the centre, she was less capable, less knowledgeable, and so on, when it came to dealing with the children. Sometimes, if a child were upset, "day staff" like me would stay late until the child was asleep, because it was generally understood that "night staff" did not have the skills to deal with the children when they were upset. They did not do counselling and they did not do restraints, so one of us had to be around if there might be a need for either. The difference between night and day was a hierarchical one: we were more skilled and competent. Although I was friendly with the night staff, and was only hired on as day staff because of my gender, it never occurred to me that there might be alternative ways of understanding this. But what this former night staff told me during our visit was that she did not feel too *incompetent* to restrain children. She was, rather, ethically opposed to it. She said something like: "you day staff: a child cries and you go in and tell them to stop or we'll lock you up. Children were sometimes upset at night after all of you left. We read to them, or just sat with them, or got them a cup of milk. That's what you do when children are upset. You care for them. You don't threaten to lock them up. When any of you heard about it, all you could say is: they're manipulating you, don't be so soft. But that's what you do when kids are upset." These are responses I would much prefer if I were upset, and it is certainly what I would want for my son if he were, which invites all sorts of reconsideration of the ways we made sense of parents and families. But sticking with the issue of restraint and ethical navigation, night staff never had to restrain children, because of what they did when children were upset, she said – implying that we had to because of what we did in initial response to the children being upset. I think this significantly influenced my decision to leave the job, although I wasn't sure I agreed with her. The very possibility that she *could* believe it shook me up. And I was very surprised by her anger about it. Why was she angry about how I was with the children? I was great with them. I thought everyone knew that.

And then there was a woman who, in the three years I worked there, was the single person who clearly conscientiously objected to physical restraints. On her first day, we restrained one of the children. She wasn't involved, but I knew that witnessing it would have been disturbing to her, so I approached her to "debrief," again depoliticizing her response as psychological and requiring correction, rather than ethical or political. She gathered up her belongings and said, "That was horrible. I can't do this," and she left, tears in her eyes.

I recall that staff mobilized non-professional discourses of psychopathology – "not right," "not healthy enough," "too emotional," and similar phrases in order to contain this person's response as aberrational and about *her*, rather than about what we had done. Perhaps we could not use terms from the professional psychologies – which we used liberally in other contexts – because this would raise questions about how she got hired in the first place, which might even unsettle the normal/abnormal binary that we needed in order to feel okay about restraining and confining other people's children. So she was narrated as occupying an interesting informal middle category that people seem to use to situate abnormality within the margins of normality and yet outside of professional intervention: phrases such as "nervous breakdown" or "not right." The implication was something like this: maybe she just had to work on her positive self-talk or her deep breathing, or even see a private therapist, and maybe then she would be healthy enough to restrain children.

One day a friend who worked in a very different social services setting walked me to the centre. One of the children hung out of his window to happily greet me and, in front of this friend, I "directed him" to go back into his room, knowing that he was surely in his room for some disciplinary reason and should not be hanging out of the window or generally enjoying himself. My friend was shocked at how I spoke to him. The Chris who had so carefully crafted his professional "adult/child boundaries," Chris the "child care counsellor," was not the Chris she knew. And again, I found the anger directed at me, her anger for how I had spoken to a child, very disruptive of my sense of what was what. I had already set my departure in motion, but this certainly heightened my sense that things were not right. And I knew as soon as I drove away from that city, with complete certainty, that I would never do those things again.

ALTERNATIVE ACCOUNTS, ETHICS, AND ACCOUNTABILITY IN THE SOCIAL WORK CLASSROOM

So what does this all have to do with what I do today in social work classrooms? I will briefly outline one example here.[7] I designed and taught a full-year history of social work course at Dalhousie University, in which I centred historical accounts about the helping professions told from the perspectives of groups that are overrepresented as non-voluntary clients. I want students to be able to perceive their future clients' protests as something other than proof of our necessity and benevolence. If a child says "you're ruining my life," I want them to think of the various histories we have read in which at times well-intentioned experts and professionals really did ruin people's lives. To this end, we read First Nations, anti-racist, mad movement, prison abolitionist, and disability studies histories of professional helping, as well as reflexive critical accounts of these histories written by helping professionals.

But what I also try to do in this course is have students generate what Michael White called a "territory of preferred identity" (2004b, 2006) from which to situate themselves in these critiques. This involves encouraging them to relate to how the histories resonate in their own lives – not so differently from what I've done here with Arendt's Eichmann – both in relation to the ways that they might have lived some aspects of their life in the margins, as members of oppressed communities, and also in relation to the privileges that they embody or, at the very least, will embody as a paid professional social worker, and perhaps in the ways that these two intersect – along the lines of my particular manifestation of what I experienced as an "alternative" masculinity playing a role in obscuring my recognition of my role in colonial, adultist, and disablist domination. Creating this "territory of preferred identity" is, I believe, what made it possible for me to write this exploration of my own perpetration of violence against disabled Aboriginal children. I can inhabit an ethical and political territory that is clear about restraints and locked confinement being wrong, which allows me to explore *how* I was so clear about it being right – or rather alright even if "unfortunate." Writing this was not easy for me to do, but I am now able to perceive the associated discomfort as a political aspect of my life. I choose to attend to such discomfort in this way, rather than psychologically, which allows me greater options in terms of what to do ethically and politically with it, in part because it allows me to reflect upon it from a territory of preferred identity rather than from a sense that something is individually wrong with me. It is this increased awareness of options that I hope to facilitate amongst my students.

CONCLUSION

Whether or not there ought to be some people in our communities who are paid to be "helpers" is an important question, although it is one that I have not touched upon. But likely there will continue to be professional helpers. And as long as there are (and likely even if we were to abolish this particular hierarchical structure), those who help need to be aware of the likelihood that we will also harm. We need to become better at becoming ethical and accountable, both when those who we are supposedly helping tell us that we are doing harm, and also when our own consciences do. My hope for this paper is that it might assist others in this process of becoming ethical.

NOTES

1 See Ahmed (1998, 2004, 2006), Arendt (1964), Butler (2004), Chapman (2007, 2009, 2010b), Derrida (1995), Fellows and Razack (1998), Foucault (1994, 2006), Goodrum, Umberson, and Anderson (2001), Hatzfeld (2005), Heron (2007), Jenkins (1990, 2009), Mahmood (2005), Neu and Therrien (2003), and Wood (2004).

2 See also Chrisjohn, Young, and Mauran 2006; and Davis 2007, for the ways that this continues to obscure power relations.

3 Brenda LeFrançois (2013) offers the following definition of adultism: "Adultism is understood as the oppression experienced by children and young people at the hands of adults and adult-produced/adult-tailored systems. It relates to the socio-political status differentials and power relations endemic to adult-child relations. Adultism may include experiences of individual prejudice, discrimination, violence, and abuse as well as social control and systemic oppression. At an individual level, it is characterized by adult authoritarianism toward children and adult-centric perspectives in interacting with children and in understanding children's experiences. Systemic adultism is characterised by adult-centric legislation, policies, rules, and practices that are imbedded within social structures and institutions which impact negatively on children's daily lives and result in disadvantage and oppressive social relations." In the treatment centre, adultism was inseparable from colonialism, disablement, and classism – although teasing them apart analytically can be somewhat useful. For example, the four oppressions each work to render the institution and its violences natural, inevitable, and so on. If our adultism was called into question, classist or colonial notions of bad parenting could explain why our control and violence was necessary, benevolent, and politically neutral with these particular children. If the colonial racism of our intervention was called into question, disablism or adultism could serve to erase race from the equation – but again always with an individualizing pathologizing gesture that rendered the children's confinement and subjection to violence exceptional. We would not want our children to be treated this way, but these children are exceptions. Indian Residential Schools were colonial and violent for aiming to segregate all Aboriginal children from their communities, but with these particular children there is no other option.

4 On this last point, see also Ahmed (2006) for a critique that may also pertain to my project.

5 "Nonviolent Crisis Intervention Training Program," Crisis Prevention Institute, Inc. (2010), http://www.crisisprevention.com/program/nci.html. Last accessed 10 October 2012.

6 "Belief Statement and Position Paper," Citizens against Restraint (2006), http://www.citizensagainstrestraint.ca/. Last accessed 10 October 2012.

7 Although I describe another aspect of this course in Chapman 2011, and describe a social work ethics course motivated by these same concerns and ideas in Chapman 2010b.

3

The Withering Away of Psychiatry: An Attrition Model for Antipsychiatry

BONNIE BURSTOW

> Of all tyrannies, a tyranny sincerely exercised for the good of its victims
> may be the most oppressive ... The robber baron's cupidity may some-
> times sleep, his cupidity may at some point be satiated, but those who tor-
> ment us for our own good torment us without end for they do so with the
> approval of their own conscience ... Their very kindness stings with intol-
> erable insult. To be "cured" against one's will and cured of states that we
> may not regard as disease is to be put on a level with those who have
> never reached the age of reason and those who never will.
>
> C.S. Lewis 1970, 292

For over 35 years, I have been an antipsychiatry activist. While the
quotation above is one with which I think that all of our community can agree, and so one that I wanted to start with, this analysis
more specifically comes out of that antipsychiatry background and
perspective. Antipsychiatry is a very particular perspective. It dif-
fers from the perspective of many people who critique psychiatry,
which is just fine, for a vibrant movement needs multiple perspectives and the fact that so many perspectives are represented in this
book is encouraging. To be clear, antipsychiatry – the perspective
from which I speak – is not one that I ask be adopted, or expect
to be adopted, by fellow radicals in this area who hold diverging
views. The point is, we form a community – the community of
people who unite to combat psychiatry. It is a wonderful community, a vibrant community. Our community encompasses differences, and we need those differences. We need all of us – antipsychiatry

activists, mad activists, professionals, survivors, artists – if we are to bring about the life-enhancing, more tolerant society toward which we are all striving.

It is critical that this be clear from the outset. One error that has tended to plague our community, as indeed it plagues almost every social movement, is that we have often fallen into vilifying others in the community with different perspectives, which is not good, or tried to convert each other, which is also not good. The fact is that we are not each other's worst enemy. The fact is that there is far more that unites us than divides us, and we need to hold onto that. The fact is, trying to convert each other is not what good allies do. My hope and trust is that we can be good allies – that we will work together where we can and in what ways we can, and where we cannot, that we will agree to take a pass, but that we will do so respectfully – that we will do so, that is, while preserving our relationships so that on all sorts of other fronts we can continue to work together.

None of this means that people who are part of particular constituencies should not try to develop their perspectives. That, in fact, is precisely what I am trying to do. I am using this chapter to flesh out a model for one such constituency – the antipsychiatry constituency. I do so because I believe in the importance of the antipsychiatry agenda. I do so because at the moment, I see this constituency as in trouble, and as far as I am concerned we need all of our community to be at the top of their game. As I look over our diverse community and how it has operated over the last couple of decades, I would have to say, I see greater clarity and greater progress in other constituencies. For some time antipsychiatry *per se* has been floundering.

One reason it is floundering no doubt is precisely because it has not always been respectful of other parts of our community. And I would like to believe that those days are over. It is floundering more significantly because the powers lined up against it are becoming increasingly stronger, increasingly more entrenched. The power of psychiatry, its continual growth, its ever more tenacious entrenchment in the state is a brutal reality and not one for which we bear responsibility. I would like to suggest, however, that antipsychiatry is also floundering because it has no model or models to guide its action.

The point is, antipsychiatry is not a new movement or constituency. A movement can proceed quite nicely for a long time fueled by passion, sincerity, vision, and ever-sharper critiques. If that sufficed

to win the battle, however, we would have succeeded long ago for
we have always had such attributes in abundance.

There comes a time, moreover, when not only does that not suf-
fice, you start to move backward. That is the nature of movements.
You have successes for a while. You have successes even without
being shrewd activists. You have successes almost no matter what
you hitch your wagon to – the politics of compassion, for example,
or the politics of entitlement like the ones associated, say, with
human rights battles. And I know because I have had such successes
– I have been there, and done that. However, inevitably the people
in power who have something to lose by your winning push back
with all the strength that their position affords them. And when they
do, that is when you need to learn how to be really good activists.
Correspondingly, that is when you absolutely need to bring something to the table to help guide action. That is the ultimate purpose
of this chapter. That is, it is to start fleshing out the beginnings of a
much-needed model for guiding antipsychiatry.

Before I go any further, I know that some people are not exactly
sure what I mean by "antipsychiatry" and are not exactly sure what
makes an antipsychiatry perspective different than the various other
perspectives which inform this book. As those differences play a
pivotal role in the model, it is critical that I clarify.

All of us who have contributed to this book are profoundly
unhappy with psychiatry. If we were not, we would not have become
involved in penning this anthology. What distinguishes an antipsychiatry stance is not simply that it is critical of psychiatry. It is that
its adherents hold that psychiatry is unqualifiedly untenable, untenable as it stands today, untenable even if it improved itself substantially. To put this another way, what distinguishes antipsychiatry
from other critical positions is the conviction that critiques of psychiatry are sufficiently conclusive, compelling, foundational, and
damning to render psychiatry as an institution inherently undesirable and irredeemable (see Burstow 2006b).

This position arises from the bitter experiences of survivors and
their writings – writings that go back to *Madness Network News*,
Phoenix Rising, and which continue to this day. More formidably,
the unqualified rejection inherent in the antipsychiatry position rests
on a number of foundational critiques. I will not be going into them
in depth, but they include: Szasz (1974) and Leifer (1990), who
demonstrate that the foundational philosophical and scientific

concepts of psychiatry are flawed; Breggin (1991) and Colbert (2001), who demonstrate that the treatments are intrinsically damaging; systemic thinkers like Mirowsky (1990), who demonstrate that the entire system of diagnostic categorization lacks validity and coherence; and labeling theorists like Goffman, who as far back as 1964 unmasked psychiatry as a form of social control.

The goal of antipsychiatry is quite simple – nothing less than the abolition or end of the psychiatric system. Herein lies its ultimate distinction. While people critical of psychiatry but not fully antipsychiatry may take certain kinds of changes as sufficient – the advent of informed consent; less use of drugs; a kinder, gentler industry; or diagnostic categories that are less overlapping, for example – as clarified in documents like the Coalition against Psychiatric Assault's (CAPA) fact sheet, antipsychiatry holds that no changes will be sufficient, for the institution is too flawed and dangerous simply to be tinkered with.[1]

A vital question arises from this goal. Namely: if the abolition of psychiatry, however conceived, is the goal, in light of that goal, how might antipsychiatry activists proceed? The question is far from simple. The fact remains that while a rigorous antipsychiatry position entails some type of abolitionist stance, no one should be under any illusion that any demands or well-worded critiques will suddenly lead to the closing of institutions or the cessation of damaging treatment. And in fact, demands that psychiatry be curbed in any more than a mere reformist way are themselves likely to lead to terror on the part of the general public and an increased emphasis on the myth of the dangerous mental patient, who must be kept under control by all available means. The point is that we are up against a very complex system, with huge vested interests, with the complicity of the state, and with the blessings of a fearful general public. We are also up against thousands of years of prejudice against people whose ways of thinking and processing differ from those of folk deemed "normal" – prejudice that, as theorists and members of the mad movement such as Esther (2000) correctly point out, predates the medical model and predates psychiatry, but has been made far more formidable by the veneer of science. Additionally, some who use psychiatric services are legitimately worried that without psychiatry, they will be out in the cold.

All that being the case, there will be no quick "win" on this issue. It is in this larger context that I ask: what might be used to guide action? If abolition on some level is the goal, what might be used as a model or touchstone in deciding what to do, what not to do, what to support, what not to support?

In foraging about for how to conceptualize a model, I have been reminded of a movement that has much in common with antipsychiatry – the prison abolition movement. While prison abolitionists uniformly agree that some people (a very small number) may need to be confined, and the details are still to be worked out, prison abolitionists, too, take abolition as the goal. Moreover, they too have been struggling with a situation where the general public approves of and indeed considers essential the very industry, approach, and complex machinery that the abolitionists hope to dismantle. Additionally, in their case too, the problematic institution in question is upheld by the state, and it is not going away overnight. Furthermore, in their case, too, albeit to a lesser extent, some inmates voluntarily seek out prison "services," with people, indeed, committing crimes precisely to get back behind bars.

What distinguishes the prison abolition movement is that it has long had a model. Now, indeed, it has had a number of models, but the most widely accepted one by far is called "the attrition model." The attrition model for prison abolition was spelled out as early as Knopp (1976) and has been reaffirmed and modified over the decades (e.g. West and Morris 2000). In the early ground-breaking book that announces the model, Knopp et al. state: "We have structured an attrition model as one example of a long range process for abolition. 'Attrition,' which means rubbing away or wearing down by frictions reflects, the *persistent* and *continuing* strategy necessary to diminish the function and power of prisons in our society" (62).

The attrition model as articulated here has at once united prison or penal abolitionists and given them a long-range basis on which to plan. Anyone who was ever been active in prison abolition will not fail to recognize the hallmark question that typically arises when a new action or campaign is considered: "Will it move us any closer to the long-term goal of prison abolition?"

An attrition model assumes that nothing as extensive and entrenched as the institution in question can be changed quickly, that something as ambitious as abolition takes place slowly and for the most part by attrition – by gradual but persistent rubbing away and wearing down. Correspondingly, it is predicated on the proposition that not all change that *seems* positive has the capacity to bring a movement closer to the abolitionist goal and indeed, on the contrary, some of what *looks promising* would actually undermine the long-term goal in question.

Herein lays a conceptualization that holds promise for antipsychiatry. My intent in this chapter is to do for antipsychiatry what was long ago done for prison abolition. The purpose of the chapter is to construct, articulate, and help readers make sense of the bare bones of an attrition model. In no way am I suggesting that it is the only possible model. Nor am I suggesting that an attrition model *per se* is straightforward or absolute. It is clear, however, that an unpopular movement that is at odds with the state and with prevailing hegemony as well as with a massive and entrenched industry begins at a serious disadvantage. It is further disadvantaged if it has no vision about how to move closer to the goal it espouses.

In presenting this attrition model, I am aware that my most focal audience are fellow activists who are antipsychiatry or who verge on it. What I can promise people from other constituencies, however, is: I'll not be forgetting you.

That said, we come to the model. It proceeds by questions – what I call "defining questions." While the number is somewhat arbitrary, let me propose three related questions that antipsychiatry activists operating from an attrition model need to ask when making major decisions. The first is the most pivotal question. The next two are auxiliary questions that might best be thought of as derivative of the first. The three questions are:

1 If successful, will the actions or campaigns that we are contemplating move us closer to the long-range goal of psychiatry abolition?
2 Are they likely to avoid improving or giving added legitimacy to the current system?
3 Do they avoid "widening" psychiatry's net (creating conditions which allow psychiatry to "scoop up" ever more people)?

To shed light on these, the first is the most formidable of the three for it states in general terms what the model is all about and as such gives abolitionists a quick reference point. Say that an action or campaign being considered is worthwhile on other grounds, but we have no reason to believe that its success will move us closer to the goal of abolition. In that case, someone else might take it up, but it

would not be the proper focus of abolitionists. To be clear, abolitionists may or may not choose to endorse such changes or campaigns, depending on whether or not it undermines the long run
goal among other things, but they would not become active in them.
The point is that an attrition mandate would require that only
changes that are abolitionist in nature and not merely reformist be
actively pursued.

Now looked at superficially, this guidance would appear to rule
out any actions not directly related to major changes. However, that
is far from the case. Part of the beauty of the attrition model is precisely that it is predicated on the passage of time. In other words,
time must be factored in, and certain types of minor changes, which
build over time, have the potential of shifting worldviews. For example, any action that helps de-medicalize the language used about
people who process differently than those deemed "normal," or live
in alternative realities, or are in emotional turmoil could be seen as
an abolitionist change, for if enough of the language shifted over
time, it would chip away at the impression that psychiatrists work
so hard at maintaining – that such states or ways of being are "medical issues" and hence the proper domain of doctors. The language
of the mad movement is an example of what could be supported in
this regard. While antipsychiatry activists in the past have been critical of mad language as not antipsychiatry *per se*, this model would
ask antipsychiatry activists to take another look.

The next question complicates what might have initially looked
simple: while question 1 asks, if successful, would our campaign or
intended actions move us closer to psychiatry abolition, question 2
asks: are they likely to avoid improving or giving legitimacy to the
current system?

While an offshoot of question 1, question 2 raises the bar. If a
campaign or action is likely to lend legitimacy to the current system,
it would make no sense for abolitionists to support it, for it undermines the ultimate goal. In fact, if lending legitimacy to the current
system is among the primary consequences of a given action then,
even if it is otherwise benign, it would not be sensible for an antipsychiatry group to even endorse it. Examples of activities sometimes engaged in by people who combat psychiatry that this
question would rule out are: sitting on task forces making recommendations on how to improve psychiatric institutions; taking part
in reformist agendas such as those associated with organizations

like the Mental Health Commission of Canada; taking part in any events or initiatives sponsored by psychiatry – including purely cultural ones for they too lend it legitimacy, indeed, making psychiatric facilities appear like friendly community centres – a valuable part of the life of the community.

Question 3 asks: if successful, would the actions or campaigns that we are contemplating avoid widening the net. What is meant by "widening the net"? It means allowing more and more people and more and more situations to fall under the auspices of psychiatry. Widening the net of psychiatry is tantamount to helping psychiatry grow as opposed to forcing it to wither. What is the intent of question three? The intent is that no initiative be adopted whose success carries with it the likely consequence of widening the net – that is, of placing more people or people at more times under the auspices of the psychiatric system. Correspondingly, where such initiatives originate from within the system, for the most part they should be actively resisted.

An obvious example of a campaign that would widen the net which originated from within the system was the push for community treatment orders.[2] Despite the rhetoric behind them, it was clear from the outset that community treatment orders would widen the net because they would drastically extend psychiatric control both temporally (past an inmate's release date) and spatially (extending the grasp of the hospital further into the community). Antipsychiatry activists, psychiatric survivors, and others critical of the system immediately saw what was at stake and while unsuccessful, quickly mobilized against the initiatives.

Psychiatric measures like this, which constitute obvious power grabs, fortunately are fairly easy to identify. By contrast, measures originating from within the community critical of psychiatry that *inadvertently* widen the net are not so easy to identify. Nonetheless, they too fall under the purview of this question, and while resistance would generally not be in order, for we do not obstruct our allies, they should not be supported or endorsed. An example of an action that would err in this regard is getting on the bandwagon clamoring for "mental health services" to be brought into an area when "mental health services" largely means psychiatric or services controlled by psychiatry.

Questions two and three may often prove difficult to hold onto, for they have the potential to place us at odds with what appears as progress, but this is precisely why they are important. Quite simply, they let us navigate tricky terrain. Let us say, for instance, that there is no service in a major city that offers emotional support for women who have undergone the shattering experience of giving birth to a stillborn child. The community responds by pushing for the creation of a service, and willy-nilly, it is decided that it will be psychiatric. Alternatively, let us say that there is a psychiatric service for women who have experienced stillbirth, but that the service is seen as deficient in some way, and the community begins pressuring to have that way addressed – say, to have the service in question expanded or otherwise improved. Given that services are direly needed for women facing this devastating life experience, one feels drawn to support both of these initiatives – for, on some level, progress is happening. As abolitionists, however, it is important to keep in mind that supporting such changes means (a) helping psychiatry get bigger, (b) helping psychiatry become firmly entrenched in yet another area, and indeed, helping psychiatry appear benign, and (c) placing an entire group of vulnerable women in more jeopardy from psychiatry than they were previously – for the inevitable depression could result in drugging, institutionalization, and even electroshock. Correspondingly, it essentially cedes the ground to psychiatry in yet another area, relegating any other services including self-help to becoming at best an alternative for those seen as least affected, and at worst an adjunct to psychiatry. These two questions about legitimating and broadening the basis of psychiatry help us see what we might otherwise fail to see. Difficult though it may be to hold onto the last two questions, accordingly, the questions are pivotal for they keep us from going off course.

Together, the three questions, along with a knowledge of how psychiatry operates, suggest obvious directions for abolitionists. What goes beyond that, they also provide antipsychiatry with one way of prioritizing – and let there be no mistake about it, we need to prioritize for we cannot do everything.

How does one prioritize using these questions? In a nutshell, the method is as follows: assume that the action or campaign being considered will be successful or at least reasonably successful, then evaluate from there. The closer to abolition some actions or directions would bring us, short of there being other objections to them, or reasons to prioritize other campaigns, the more focal they should be to antipsychiatry organizing. Correspondingly, anything that actually attacks psychiatry's power base is particularly important and, so should be given top priority.

To spell out what some of those top priority actions, directions, or campaigns might be – and people familiar with the terrain will recognize most of these – particularly apropos and indeed, more central than they are currently, would be actions or campaigns that put the state on the defensive when it comes to psychiatry or weakens the state's unilateral endorsement or funding of psychiatry. The reason why this direction is singularly important is the pivotal role of the state in psychiatric rule. Psychiatry has the power it does only because it is an extension of the state, is part of the apparatus of the state, and as such, is additionally handsomely funded by the state. Loosen the tie with the state, eliminate all or a sizable part of the state's sanction or support, and psychiatry's size and power to harm begins to evaporate.

Examples of actions or campaigns that might be taken up in this regard – and most of these have long figured in our community arsenal – include: directly suing the state for damages; suing hospitals for damages; challenging the constitutionality of laws that the state has enacted to empower psychiatry; appealing to a power outside the state, whether it be the UN or some other international body. I give kudos here to the work of people like David Oaks. Other less foundational but also critically important measures on the same continuum include: demanding moratoriums on new psychiatric hospital constructions; pressuring for the end to involuntary commitment; initiatives that support increased patients' rights or the upholding of current rights; advocating cutbacks in funding for psychiatric services and increased funding for more benign services; waging campaigns to de-fund private psychotherapy delivered by doctors, or what I think might well serve us better, to fund equally psychotherapy delivered by others (psychiatry could not have the power which it has today without the state giving it a virtual monopoly).

Many of the other initiatives that survivors and other critics of psychiatry commonly take up would also be focal. Included, in this regard, would be consciousness-raising, for consciousness-raising can also clearly help us, as a society, move toward attrition. Included are attacks on other parts of the psychiatric industrial complex – not the least of which are the pharmaceutical companies upon which psychiatry fundamentally rests. Foundational critiques – that is, critiques of the basic tenets underpinning psychiatric practice – are particularly important.

By the same token, actions that are abolitionist in nature with respect to any of the current "treatments" can be seen as in line with the abolitionist agenda. This, of course, would include the rigorously abolitionist campaigns currently waged by heroic survivors and their allies to ban electroshock (for more detail, see Weitz 2008). Nevertheless, it would also include actions, campaigns, and recommendations that are not immediately abolitionist with respect to current treatment, but which are likely (if successful) to contribute to attrition. An example is a number of the recommendations put forward in a report submitted by a panel that oversaw Toronto-based hearings into psychiatric drugs in 2005. None of the recommendations in the report were abolitionist in the immediate sense of the term. If enacted, however, most would further the long-term work of attrition.

Take, for example, the recommendation "all doctors who prescribe psychiatric drugs be required by law to review the choice of drugs and the amount of the drug administered ... doctors in particular be required biannually to consider less powerful drugs, drugs with less negative effects ... smaller doses, and withdrawal itself." (Burstow, Cohan, Diamond et al. 2005). Clearly, if measures such as these were enacted, they would contribute to the weakening of psychiatry and the gradual loosening of the psychiatric drug stranglehold. Note, in this regard, that besides the fact that any substantial loosening of the drug stranglehold is desirable in and of itself, in addition psychiatry's claim to jurisdiction over madness lies largely with the drugs. Any attack on the drugs is, in the long run, an attack on psychiatry's relevance.[3]

Many, albeit not all, of the examples articulated so far are obvious. What is particularly useful about an attrition model, however, is that it helps activists and analysts engage in the reasoning, weighing, and balancing needed when confronted with choices that are not at all obvious, or what is not uncommon, where disagreement arises. And such guides are essential to better functioning.

To offer a practical example of how attrition-type reasoning helped an antipsychiatry group work through a difficult and contentious issue, I would highlight a situation that arose recently in CAPA. A request came from a member-at-large to endorse a bill most everyone here is aware of – the New York bill banning involuntary electroshock on children under sixteen.[4] As the request came during the summer when CAPA was not meeting, it fell to the executive to decide. Initially, the CAPA executive was seriously split. Initially, most of the executive did not want to endorse because CAPA's own position is the complete abolition of electroshock, also because they feared that any new law of this nature would lend legitimacy to electroshock. On the other hand, the rest of the executive and the member-at-large were convinced that the initiative should be endorsed because if such legislation were passed, it would stop some people from being electroshocked, also because it moves in the direction of the abolition of shock.

To be clear, this dispute predates any articulation of an attrition model for antipsychiatry. Attrition, nonetheless, was at issue from the beginning, and it is a careful focusing on attrition that allowed this question to be resolved. *One* of the reasons given against endorsing drew on a principle inherent in the attrition model – that such a new law would lend legitimacy to the electroshock industry. *All* of the reasons to endorse connected with attrition principles: that is, it prevents some people from being electroshocked, or to put it another way, would narrow the electroshock net. Additionally, it would begin chipping away at electroshock. The point is, if electroshock is not good for children, it could be argued, it is also not good for the elderly. Accordingly, the successful passing of such a bill would take New York one stage closer to abolishing electroshock for other populations and potentially ultimately for everyone.

The principles of attrition allowed us to quickly work through what began as a divisive and hotly debated issue. It was determined that the worry that such a new law would lend credibility to the electroshock industry was ill founded. Additionally, it was agreed that such a law would protect some people, narrow the sway of electroshock, and lead in the direction of electroshock abolition. Significantly, all members of the executive followed the logic. What is also significant, none of these deliberations weakened or any way altered CAPA's own commitment to personally launch only ECT actions that call for complete abolition. However, it did allow us to work through the endorsement issue and quickly transit from a seemingly irresolvable standoff to endorsement of a bill that merited our support.

The three questions I have been discussing are the definitional ones, and indeed, are the questions that ensure that antipsychiatry initiatives are compatible with the ultimate antipsychiatry goal. This notwithstanding, given the complexity of the issues, given the vulnerability of some who access psychiatric services, and given our broader commitments as human beings, of course, these are not the only questions that antipsychiatry activists should be asking when contemplating new actions or campaigns. While it is beyond the scope of this chapter to discuss these, besides questions of strategy, additional questions that I would recommend organizations or individuals holding an attrition model ask themselves include: What sorts of non-psychiatric services, what sort of help – self help, for example, or withdrawal centres – are we advocating or supporting? Are we finding ways to link up with others in the critical of psychiatry community – psychiatric survivor organizations and mad groups in particular? Given that psychiatry is not the first oppressor of the people deemed mad, what measures are we taking to avoid helping pave the way for another oppressor to replace psychiatry?[5] Is the initiative that we are considering compatible with the creation of a more caring society? Does it leave any vulnerable people in the lurch? Does the initiative that we are considering in any way empower the people most affected or most at risk from the psychiatric system (past psychiatric patients, current psychiatric patients, people who would appear to have psychiatry on their horizon)? Are we paying sufficient attention to the special jeopardy in which psychiatry places otherwise oppressed populations? Women? People who are homeless? Racialized people? Lesbians and gays? Transsexuals – transsexual youth in particular? Arguably, most importantly of all, the elderly?[6]

As regards this last item, the point is that psychiatric oppression intersects in horrific and manifold ways with all systemic oppressions, and it is critical that it be critiqued and attacked with that awareness. Hence, the profound significance of such developments as feminist antipsychiatry, and the very particular agendas, mandates, and priorities that these open up.[7]

At this point, I have given some idea how this model can be used to determine what to actively take up and what not take up, what to support and what not support. I have also shown how it can be used to establish priorities, and what some of those priorities might be. At this juncture I want to enter trickier territory. I indicated at the beginning that use of the attrition model would inevitably lead to a re-examination of some of the types of activities that some of us would have supported in the past, and I want to touch on some of the areas where the model would encourage rethinking. One such area is certain measures taken up – and understandably taken up – with regard to different oppressions.

Notwithstanding the enormous importance of paying rigorous attention to systemic oppression and notwithstanding the legitimacy of differing priorities, there have long been initiatives related to oppressed groups that an attrition model require be looked at more critically. These include: pressuring for the removal of specific noxious diagnoses that particularly or uniquely oppress members of an otherwise oppressed group, and advocating for culturally sensitive psychiatric services.

First, critiquing specific diagnoses is not only unproblematic, it is a critical part of consciousness-raising, on which all attrition models depend, and as such, it is mandatory for antipsychiatry. Indeed, targeting specific diagnoses has quite rightly been one of the hallmarks of feminist antipsychiatry. Whether as women, or as racialized people, or both, we want the damage done to our communities acknowledged and stopped. Correspondingly, oppressed populations have ample reason to want specific diagnoses removed from the books that uniquely pathologize these particular populations and make it easy for psychiatry to intrude. Included, in this regard, are such historical diagnoses as "ego-dystonic homosexuality" and "hysterical personality disorder" (currently "histrionic personality disorder"), which have oppressed the lesbian and gay and the women's community respectively, and current diagnoses as "gender identity disorder," which are oppressive to the trans community.[8]

That women, lesbians and gays, and trans people work to have such diagnoses quashed is hardly surprisingly. The primary question here is not whether women, gays and lesbians, or trans people should organize against such diagnoses, or even whether people generally critical of psychiatry should organize against them. It is whether or not mobilization against such diagnoses is a proper antipsychiatry initiative. Herein the attrition model sheds its own light, albeit I have no questions that intersecting identities make this issue particularly complicated for many.

Ultimately, for an attritionist, the issue at hand boils down to: How does the existence of a campaign against one or other diagnosis measure up to the definitional questions? That is, do the successes of such campaigns contribute to the erosion of psychiatry? Do they avoid widening the net? And do they avoid improving or lending legitimacy to psychiatry? Now the question of widening the net is unclear. However, enough of these campaigns have "succeeded" to demonstrate that there are no encouraging answers to the other questions. A number of diagnoses that we, as women, and as lesbians and gays, rightly find oppressive have been struck down – and yet these successes have not impeded psychiatry, changed it significantly, or resulted in fewer diagnoses. On the contrary, the number of diagnoses continues to skyrocket (see Kirk and Kutchins 1992, 1994). Given psychiatry's ingenuity in hiding old unpopular diagnoses behind new labels (for a discussion of this tendency, see Burstow 1990), and given its ability to turn acknowledged oppression into a syndrome, it is often unclear what is achieved for the actual population in question. At best, the new diagnoses constitute somewhat of an improvement, albeit not the kind that contributes to attrition; and at worst, they only appear to improve, drawing people who began as critical into their terrain in the process. What is also problematic, such campaigns give legitimacy to psychiatry for they tacitly acknowledge its authority by the sheer act of appealing to it. Moreover, the apparent success of such campaigns has lent psychiatry the further credibility of allowing it to appear progressive. As such, involvement in such campaigns is questionable for abolitionists, although progressive professionals with antipsychiatry leanings such as Caplan have long engaged in them, and continued discussion is important.[9]

A similar problem arises with respect to campaigns for more culturally sensitive psychiatric approaches – and, what is particularly problematic, for the creation of new culturally sensitive psychiatric programs. Again, it is totally understandable that populations affected by psychiatric racism, or sexism, or transphobia would push for such changes. And given the dearth of funding for services not under the auspices of psychiatry, it is totally understandable that communities that are not mainstream – especially those subject to significant transgenerational trauma and/or insidious trauma – would ask for the creation of culturally sensitive psychiatric programs, whether it be the trans community or the Aboriginal communities.[10] Nonetheless, such campaigns are in conflict with all three major tenets of an attrition model: they do not move us closer to abolition; they do not avoid improving or lending legitimacy to the current system – in fact they are precisely reformist changes, which serve to improve psychiatry and give it greater credibility; and they widen the net, allowing more and more members of the populations in question to fall under psychiatric auspices, and now with the active cooperation of their community. As such, campaigns for such services are at odds with psychiatry abolition and arguably hazardous for the communities in question.

If an attrition model became a standard part of an antipsychiatry toolkit, inevitably, other types of mobilization that currently may look benign or like a reasonable trade off would likewise start looking increasingly problematic or minimally incompatible with an abolition mandate. The question would be to weigh carefully, to be open to reconsidering, to factor in other questions as needed – and what is particularly important, to understand that allies who make different decisions remain our allies.

Throughout this chapter, I have been demonstrating how an attrition model can help antipsychiatry activists make choices, establish priorities, and rethink directions and initiatives. While I do not suggest that is equal, in ending, I would like to suggest that there is something in this model for other constituencies in our community as well. Now I do not wish to overstate my hand here, for it could sow division as well. If applied sensitively, this model might nonetheless be of assistance in easing some of the tension between antipsychiatry activists and others in our community and in creating bridges. It might foster clearer communication and understanding, for example. Additionally, it might enable antipsychiatry organizations to support and join with others in more initiatives.

Significantly, while not identified as antipsychiatry, many of the initiatives, focuses, and actions specific to other critical constituencies have the potential of whittling away at psychiatry, and as such, could be supported by the antipsychiatry community far more enthusiastically than they have been in the past. An example is the creation and defense of a mad culture – Mad Pride events, articulations of mad theory – which to date, sadly, has received little support from antipsychiatry. The attrition model provides a way of recognizing points of meeting that are obscured by other types of abolitionist stances, for these become visible when approached from the vantage point of slow but persistent wearing away. It also provides others in the larger community with a view of what might be added or what modifications might be made to turn an action inimical to antipsychiatry into one that antipsychiatry groups can actively support or minimally endorse. While I would not wish to overstate the case, the model also might be of more direct assistance to the broader activist community. The point is, while other constituencies legitimately have other priorities – and I am speaking particularly to activists who organize in relation to psychiatry here – I can see the value of groups with different perspectives engaging with the attrition model from time to time.

Bottom line: those of us who organize in this area have this in common: None of us are deliriously happy with psychiatry. All of us minimally would like it smaller, would like it curtailed, would like room for more benign help to take root. In other words, all constituencies in our community in some way favour some type of withering. Accordingly, groups with other perspectives may be served by at least occasionally having these three questions among the ones they consider when choosing actions or campaigns.

In conclusion, I invite others to come up with their own models and to share them, whether they be models for antipsychiatry, models for the mad movement or models for the psych survivor movement. The reality is, we need a plethora of workable models if we are to bring about the more caring, tolerant society for which we are all fighting. And let there be no mistake about it. Besides that they have the lion's share of the power, people who successfully make this world a living hell for others – who rob others of their freedom, who subject them to torturous treatments – tend to be very good at what they do. *We* need to be equally good.

NOTES

1 In 2008 CAPA created a myth/fact sheet to correct misimpressions about antipsychiatry, as well as to help bring the community together. For CAPA's Antipsychiatry Fact Sheet, see http://coalitionagainstpsychiatri cassault.wordpress.com/fact-sheet/./mental-health/ brief-psychotherapy-centre-for-women-%28bpcw%29463/.

2 For an insightful critique of community treatment orders as well as a compelling read, see Fabris (2006).

3 For a highly informative exploration of the role of psychiatric drugs in entrenching and propping up psychiatric power, see Scull (1977).

4 Sponsored by Assemblyman Ortiz, the bill may be found at http://assembly. state.ny.us/leg/?bn=A08779&sh=t.

5 Earlier oppressors include the church and businessmen. See, in this regard, Szasz (1977).

6 For an examination of the special jeopardy of oppressed populations, see Breggin (1991) and Burstow (2003). For an examination of the massive psychiatrization of the elderly and its tragic effects, see Breggin (1991). For a revealing look at ageism in the administration of electroshock, see Weitz (1997).

7 See, in this regard, Blackbridge and Gilhooly (1985); Burstow (2003); Chan, Chunn, and Menzies (2005); Chesler (1972); Grobe (1995); and Smith (1987).

8 For a discussion of various diagnoses that have historically served, or currently serve, to pathologize people from the L G B T Q community, see Burstow (1990). For a discussion of diagnoses oppressive to women, see Unger (2004) and Caplan (1995). For the articulation of the diagnosis gender identity disorder, see D S M - I V - T R (American Psychiatric Association, 2000, 576ff.).

9 For Caplan's own account of her involvement in this regard, see Caplan (1995).

10 Transgenerational trauma is trauma passed down from one generation to the next. Insidious trauma is the everyday trauma of living in a world in which you are oppressed. For further elaboration on these terms, see Burstow (2003).

4

Psychology Politics Resistance: Theoretical Practice in Manchester

IAN PARKER

This chapter teases out principles and dynamics associated with a particular moment of resistance that went by the name of "Psychology Politics Resistance" and occurred in Manchester in the 1990s, and which bears a special relationship to psychology. While not explicitly targeting psychiatry, the chapter figures in this book on resistance to psychiatry because psychology is not an isolated practice or domain of thought but part of what is commonly called the psy-complex (Rose 1996). Included in this complex are psychiatry, psychology, and psychotherapy, and by extension, psychiatric social work and psychiatric nursing. As the various elements within the psy-complex are intricately related, resistance within or with respect to one element necessarily has implications for resistance by or with respect to the others. What is equally significant, this moment in Manchester was a historically important moment of resistance.

The campaigning group "Psychology Politics Resistance" (PPR) was part of a wave of radical activity in and against the discipline of psychology in the 1990s. Following its founding conference in Manchester in 1994 the group published six newsletters, and its members were involved in a number of different campaigns before it effectively dissolved itself into *Asylum: Magazine for Democratic Psychiatry* (which still incorporates the PPR Newsletter).[1] This chapter reviews the specific cultural-economic conditions of the 1990s that facilitated and hindered the development of the group, explores the assumptions it made about what was possible and the rationale for the name, and draws out theoretical and practical lessons. P P R, or something very like it, is just as necessary today, if not more so, and this account is also designed to stimulate the rebirth of the group. We will begin with the "time" of P P R.

WHY PPR THEN?

The founding conference of "Psychology Politics Resistance" in Manchester on 2 July 1994 was the culmination of a series of meetings of radicals in the U K dissatisfied with the discipline of psychology from the mid 1980s. The founding 150-strong conference was deliberately international in character, and included guest speaker contributions from a psychologist working in the prison system in Barcelona (Pep Garcia-Borés); a psychologist active in the struggle against apartheid in South Africa (Don Foster); and an educational psychologist (Snezana Frzina) from Sarajevo then in exile in Manchester as a result of the civil war. A collection was taken for the campaign support group "Workers Aid for Bosnia." Key to the thinking of P P R was that it needed to draw together three different kinds of networks. Academics who taught and researched psychology, and who were mainly based in psychology departments, were at the core of the group, and they used their institutional resources to build meetings and distribute campaign materials, including the P P R newsletters.[2]

These academics were reluctant to take a lead, however, and made an initial alliance with professional psychologists who saw firsthand the problematic nature of the different models and treatments offered by the discipline. These two networks, academic and professional, then sought to make a further alliance with groups of what are sometimes called "users," sometimes "consumers," and sometimes "survivors" of psychology services. These labels are each inaccurate, and either reclaimed or avoided by different groups. It is this third part of the alliance – those who suffer firsthand what psychology does, and speak out against the discipline – that was the heart and conscience of P P R. A guest speaker, Ron Coleman, at the founding conference, for example, was from the Hearing Voices Network and *Asylum: Magazine for Democratic Psychiatry*. In this sense, the decision to fold the P P R newsletter into *Asylum* at the time of the re-launch of the magazine in 2002 (one of its many "re-launches," it should be said) was a logical step. That decision marked the end of an eight-year span of life for P P R in its first incarnation, and it is worth reflecting for a moment on the context of that existence, then, in order to understand something about its specific "conditions of possibility."

One reason the founding conference was "international" was because we knew already that the cultural-economic climate at home – in Manchester and in the UK – was a difficult one, and that we needed to maintain connections with like-minded colleagues in other countries if we were to survive. After the election of Margaret Thatcher at the head of the Conservative Party in 1979, psychology was the site of an immense ideological assault by the ruling class as it sought to roll back the post-Second World War welfare state and throw the population into the maelstrom of neoliberal economic policies. Those were early days of this assault, one that has become significantly more intense since the capitalist economic crisis and the securitization agenda of the state to deal with dissent.

It is possible to see more clearly now that neoliberalism – a transformation of capitalism that privatizes collectively held resources, and demands that each individual configures themselves as a resilient flexible entrepreneur of their own selves willing to adapt to changing market conditions – required *more* psychology. The neoliberal turn has a particular impact on women, and all the more so when the service sector in nations within the global north becomes the fastest-growing part of the economy. And in many other nations in the global south, the service sector, which has a high proportion of female employees, is also now the dominant sector of the economy. This is a continuation of a mutation of capitalism into so-called "late capitalism" that began with an electronic "third industrial revolution" after the Second World War, and which entails a globalization of production and consumption (Mandel 1974). The service sector relies on stereotypical women's abilities to resonate with the needs of others. Women as caregivers and centres of emotional support are harnessed by the service sector – in restaurants, hotels, and leisure facilities as well as in "customer care" and personnel departments of large companies – in the form of "emotional labour" (Hochschild 1983).

This means that not only is the family still effectively a kind of prison for many women – idealized as the place where all should be safe at home in the care of women but often a place of silent misery where the power of the man is allowed to actually govern its internal structure – but it is no longer sealed off as any kind of haven from the outside world (Zaretsky 1976). Women are expected to be as busy ministering to the needs of others in their workplace as they are at home, and the "emotional labour" they undertake leads to deeper and more draining forms of alienation. Women, and the men who learn from them how to behave nicely to customers and clients at work, are thus expected to engage more fully in their work and the stage is set for more pressure and more personal breakdowns for those who are eventually unable to cope. Even in the early 1980s academic psychologists could see a consequence of this neoliberal turn; the discipline of psychology became much more popular as people were ideologically corralled into finding individual solutions to the problems they faced, and came to believe that "psychology" itself was one of those solutions.

On the left too there was disenchantment with a political-economic explanation of the crisis, and there were attempts to understand "Thatcherism" as a specific cultural-ideological phenomenon that called upon some kind deep-seated psychological investment in authority. Some therapist-activists even sought to revive Wilhelm Reich's psychoanalytic writings on the mass psychology of fascism in the 1930s and use a version of those ideas to explain the mass psychology of Thatcherism (Chaplin and Haggart 1983). Other radical academics looked to a combination of psychoanalysis and "post-structuralist" theory to account for the "new times" we faced, and this ethos underpinned the work of one of the influential radical psychology journals *Ideology and Consciousness* (that ran from 1977–81) and then the path-breaking book *Changing the Subject* (Henriques et al. 1984) published a few years later. By that time the terms "ideology" and "consciousness" had themselves became embarrassing reminders of an attachment to what they saw as old-style Marxist and feminist politics, and shortly before its demise *Ideology and Consciousness* was abbreviated to "*I & C*."

The deep disappointment with the failure of the left in the 1970s led many activists into psychotherapy, and a good proportion of those into training as counsellors, psychotherapists, or psychoanalysts themselves. This meant that even at the moment of an intensification of appeals to "psychology" under Thatcher, there was likewise a retreat into some kind of psychology by those who knew that something was deeply wrong with this retreat into the interior of the individual. It is in that context, in those "conditions of possibility" that a small group (Erica Burman, Corinne Squire) who had been inspired by the critique of psychology developed in *Changing the Subject* set up small group meetings to discuss the ideas in the book. And it is in that context that we found ourselves complaining about a discipline that was increasing in strength and visibility in culture around us. One of the uncomfortable paradoxes of those times was that because higher education institutions were keen to expand their market-share, they were also willing to tolerate the work of young critical academics wanting to put on conferences and short courses on what was wrong with psychology. Up until the 1980s we would have been closely scrutinized concerning the content of such activities, and asked whether this was genuinely part of psychology. From that moment, however, the only question the colleges and universities were asking was how many people could be recruited to take part and, if at all possible, how much money they would bring in.

WHAT IS IN THE NAME?

The name we chose was to be punctuated, concluded with the term "resistance." Why? First we need to step back and understand something about the nature of signifiers, for example "resistance." Signifiers are elements of meaning, the material inscription of meaning in what the linguist Ferdinand de Saussure (1974) called the "sound image." The concept we each attach to the sound image or signifier "resistance" will be different, but an important factor that links the concepts we might have with each other, and which makes collective meaning-making and political activity possible, is that the meaning of a signifier is given by its relation with other terms. It is that relation we had to weigh up when choosing how to name our group.

We had earlier meetings in the late 1980s in London and Manchester (and there were similar meetings in other cities in the UK) under the name "Changing the Subject," for example, but this phrase seemed too closely tied to an academic psychology book – an internal scholarly argument – and a bit too playful and cryptic for us. Anyway, for those who are on the sharp end of psychology, is not the discipline always trying to "change" them as subjects, to make them adapt to what the discipline wants them to be? By 1989 we opted for a much broader accessible name "Psychologists for Social Justice and Equality" (PSJE), and we got as far as setting out

a "general basis," "aims and objectives," and an outline of "organization and activities" (which specified that there should be four
coordinators and that there would be a "differential" in membership
subscription prices between waged and unwaged). Looking back at
this now, I am struck by how bureaucratic it looks, and it seems to
combine in its name a well-meaning liberal ethos with the assumption that everyone involved would be "psychologists." It is then
entirely understandable that PSJE should state (in its "general
basis") that it would be "committed to developing psychological
ideas" and that it wanted "psychology to change from a conservative into an openly liberatory discipline."

There were two practical-theoretical steps we needed to take.
One was to see that such a group needed to dislodge the priority
given in the name PSJE to "psychologists." Surely the fact that
psychologists were telling other people how to behave and think
was precisely the problem, and this problem would not be resolved
by us telling people that they ought to be in favour of "social justice
and equality." In other words, we had to realise that there is a difference between an ethical stance we might take in relation to the
discipline – an ethical stance of "resistance," as we came to name
it – and the suffocating "moral" standpoint which tried to get people to conform to what we thought was right. Morality specifies
what is right and what is wrong, and operates as a series of codes
to which people should adjust themselves. Ethics, on the other
hand, opens up the possibility for people to decide for themselves
and to make alliances to say no to power, and to remain faithful to
events that have changed the coordinates of taken-for-granted reality (Badiou 2001).

The second step we needed to take was to avoid the surreptitious
reintroduction of something psychological, as commonly understood, into the process of resistance itself. We took the first step with
a renaming of the group, later in 1989, as "Psychology and Social
Responsibility" (PSR), but we needed to take a second step away
from the notion of "social responsibility" itself, which I think we
can see now was a psychologized (and rather moralistic) phrase that
risked inviting people into exactly the kind of position that the psychologists would like them to adopt. That is, one of the defining
characteristics of psychology as a discipline is precisely that it aims
to turn its subjects into self-governing individuals who will take
responsibility for their own actions, as if it was all down to them,

and they are seen as pathological if they are not willing to do that
(Rose 1996).

If we reflect for a moment on "Psychology," "Politics," and
"Resistance" as signifiers, and upon "Psychology Politics Resistance"
combined as a signifier, we can see that there are some important
theoretical issues at stake (Howarth et al. 2000). First, what the
name came to mean is itself a signifying process, and it breaks usual
grammatical rules by avoiding commas between the terms or add-
ing "and" between the politics and resistance. The three words are
chained together in a quite specific way, in a relation of succession
and, almost, of equivalence. There was thus ambiguity that was not
present in the previous incarnations of the name of the group over
what the place of "psychology" was in relation to power and resistance, and certainly it did not suppose that any kind of psychology
was part of a solution or alternative to politics and resistance.

Second, we can ask what types of signifiers were mobilized in this
naming of the group. There are certain kinds of signifiers in a language that anchor meaning and in tying it down they operate as
"master signifiers." Other signifiers are more ambiguous and there
is an ideological battle over who can claim them and over what
they will mean in relation to the other signifiers around them.
These signifiers operate as what have been termed "floating signifiers." And there is a third kind of signifier, which comes to stand in
for the impossible fullness and universality of society that people fill
with their hopes and dreams for a better world, for the best possible
world – and these are "empty signifiers."

The third theoretical issue concerns the historical context, which
gives sense to terms in a language. Because the meaning or value of
terms is given by their place in a particular signifying system – language at a moment in time – we need to be able to step back and
map what these values are so that the choice we make for the name
of our group will function in such a way as to both resonate with
and contest prevailing meanings. To show how and why this is
important, let us look at what "psychology," "politics," and "resistance" have come to mean to us.

PSYCHOLOGY, POLITICS, AND RESISTANCE

PPR was sometimes given the full title "Psychology, Politics, Resistance," with commas separating the three key signifiers from each

other. The removal of the commas, to give the accurate title of the group, chains these signifiers together in a more direct way, and produces a new combined signifier. This new signifier, if my memory is right, was suggested by some colleagues (John Bowers and Liam Greenslade) who were particularly interested in the work of Michel Foucault, and they had most probably noticed the productive con-catenation of terms in books of his such as *"Language, Counter-Memory, Practice"* (Foucault 1977b) (which did even then retain the commas) and *"Power/Knowledge"* (Foucault 1980a).

Foucault had been a key point of reference for those of us reading *Changing the Subject* (Henriques et al. 1984) and organizing meetings to discuss the book. Some of Foucault's ideas about power surfaced in far-left politics in London in the wake of the "post-structuralist" and arguments from the work of the Italian Marxist Antonio Gramsci inside the "eurocommunist" Communist Party of Great Britain in which the ideas of Laclau and Mouffe (1985) were moving the party in a more rightward, social democratic direction before its eventual dissolution (Mandel 1978). A small group (Labour Briefing) inside the Labour Party attempted to push the Greater London Council further to the left – for example with the slogan "Labour – Take the Power!" (Reicher 1987). There was some small overlap between the membership of PPR and its earlier incarnations and Labour Briefing in the late 1980s. And, crucially, Foucault's *History of Madness* (2009) in its earlier, abridged, English-language version had made an impact on the user/survivor movement, and his work on surveillance and control (Foucault 1977a) resonated with those on the sharp end of psychiatry. Some of his ideas that were accompanying the debates in the left now came to augment the arguments made by activists in groups like the Mental Patients Union – groups that had always combined radical theory with practice (Spandler 2006).

PSYCHOLOGY

Foucault was a psychology instructor for several years, and a broad critique of the psy-complex that includes psychiatry, psychology, and psychotherapy haunted his writing from the book on "madness" to his last writings on the formation of the subject (Ingleby 1985). At the theoretical core of his historical investigations is the question of how the human subject in Western Enlightenment comes to fold around and reflect upon itself, how reflexivity as such begins to operate as a touchstone for how people think and act upon themselves.[3] This personal connection between theory and practice – the Kantian injunction to have the courage to think for yourself[4] – is sedimented in the discipline of psychology, which turns that ethic into a form of morality. What should be noticed now, however, is that the development of psychology out of the tradition of the Western Enlightenment is concerned with truth as an empirically verifiable system of knowledge about the nature of the human being.

"Truth" is very different in various cultural traditions, which is something the globalization of English-language forms of subjectivity (of which psychology is a key part) is now obscuring (Tazi 2004). What the discipline of psychology does is to drum in particular ideas about what it is important to know about human beings in order to educate and treat them, and – this is essential – to enforce a particular view of what that truth as such should look like. When we ask ourselves the question "What is psychology" we are therefore brought face-to-face with a fundamental question about what counts as truth, and who should do the counting (Canguilhem 1958). Psychology as a discipline aims to accumulate knowledge about the individual human being, and operates on the assumption that empirical study of behaviour is the basis for modelling internal psychological processes and so then knowing how to put them right when they have gone wrong. What psychology refuses to do is to step back and notice how its description of us as cognitive behavioural mechanisms is actually a function of capitalist society. Because it refuses to do that it turns its descriptions into prescriptions for good behaviour and correct cognition that adapt us, make us fit all the more tightly and willingly into the way the world is now (Parker 2007).

This poses a huge challenge to radical or "critical" psychologists, one that was tackled over and again in PPR, to give up their well-meaning idea that if the bad bits of the discipline were scraped off then we would be left with some good authentic descriptions of psychology that could be useful. Meetings of PPR sometimes turned into debates about what bits of the discipline could be retrieved, and we could see our colleagues at different moments attaching themselves to "community psychology," or "action research," or even psychoanalysis as a starting point for their critique of the other bits of the discipline they did not like. These apparently academic questions did, of course, have immediate implications for professional psychologists (though a group of psychologists working in the National Health Service in north Manchester we once spoke to about PPR told us that they actually had no time to do any "psychology" because they were too busy giving advice about housing rights and supporting social networks).

For sure the debates had implications for user/survivors of psychology. For them, a psychological theory could be useful, but the grounds for judging that had nothing to do with the criteria that were being used in the university departments that carried out "research" or those used in the clinics that had to meet "targets." We learned that the "good" and "bad" of psychology was always revealed in its practice, and that attempts to define what psychology really was as a starting point was a topsy-turvy way of addressing the problem. Psychology operates as a kind of master signifier that holds things in place and psychologists learn to use other master signifiers to anchor their own particular understanding of reality. Our task in PPR was to destabilize that master signifier, and open up some space for those subject to it.

POLITICS

In other words, and here the chaining of "psychology" directly to the next signifier in our name is important, the grounds on which we should assess what worked should be political. "Politics" was, for some participants in the meetings, the most contentious part of the equation. Unlike "social justice," "equality," or "social responsibility," the signifier "politics" forces us to engage with structural conditions and with the multitude of different social actors who are aiming to change the world. It goes beyond the rather vacuous earlier names which, in the words of one participant in PPR (Steve Reicher), boiled down to "psychologists against bad things."

There are two aspects of the signifier "politics" that were important to us in PPR. One aspect concerned the state, the apparatus of last resort when challenges to authority (and challenges to capitalism) become too much. Any number of complaints against abuse by psychologists or demands for fair treatment could be made that simply then result in the giving of a little more leeway to those who complain and serve to humour and shut up those who are complaining and demanding. But when the oppressed are organized in such a way that they really might change the conditions that perpetuate their oppression, we come up against the realm of the state.

The second important aspect of the signifier "politics" was connecting with the realm of what we ourselves learned to call our "psychological" being (that part of ourselves that the psychologists are supposed to have expertise in understanding and managing). This second aspect came to the fore with the development of a stronger feminist presence inside socialist politics in the 1970s, and concerns the way that everyday social relationships perpetuate wider power relations. Socialist feminism brings in an aspect of politics that is captured in the slogan "the personal is the political" (Rowbotham et al. 1980). A consequence of that way of reconfiguring the nature of politics is that our attempts to change prevailing social conditions should in the very process of change "prefigure" what we would wish for as another world (Kagan and Burton 2000). Already, then, the connection of the term "politics" with the term "psychology" produces a change in "value" or meaning of each of the terms, so that we understand the meaning of the terms "psychology" and "politics" differently.

There is a third aspect of the politics of psychology that we now need to consider, something of which we were dimly aware in the 1980s but which has become more salient now in globalized neoliberal capitalism. That is, the temptation to respond to the politics of psychology with a psychological approach to politics, and more generally with an intensification of what has been termed "psychologization" (De Vos 2012). Psychology today does not only operate as a discipline to which people are subjected when they fall out of line, but it has proliferated in everyday discourse and practices of self-monitoring and self-improvement in the media and everyday life. This "psychologization" of our ways of relating to ourselves and others is an intensification of the kind of thing Foucault (1984b) was so interested in at the birth of the Western Enlightenment, and now this intensification and regulation of subjectivity is being rolled out around the world in new forms of cultural imperialism. If the new colonial subjects want to make themselves understood they must speak about themselves in psychological terms. By articulating "psychology" with "politics" then, we thereby turn "psychology" into a "floating signifier" and give it a new meaning as we draw it across into part of our discourse, into the discourse of the oppressed, into the discourse of those who resist psychology.

RESISTANCE

Psychology is a profoundly "moral" discipline in the worst sense of the term. Like the most apparently open and enlightened versions of psychiatry, psychology wants the human subject to speak about itself, and puts a moral value on "empowerment" and "participation" of subjects in the forms of understanding and treatment that the discipline thinks it is developing. This means that "resistance" to psychology can be quickly and effectively psychologized; those who resist are thereby blamed and pathologized for their "unreasonable" behaviour and their faulty understanding of what the discipline can offer to them. The activities of PPR were designed to thwart that effort at pathologization that psychology is usually so good at, and that meant handling the question of the voice of the oppressed in a careful practical and theoretical way (McLaughlin 1996).

Hence the diversity of PPR initiatives, that included the "PPR Networks Festival 1998" (which brought together a number of allied groups, some of which we rather strongly disagreed with, a rather bruising experience). There was "The North West Right to Refuse Electroshock Campaign," which tactically put aside the question about whether electroshock worked or not and honed in on the rather more pressing issue of how those who are already vulnerable are subjected to this "treatment" against their will. We connected with other issues through the Women in PPR group and participating in the "Asylum in the 21st Century" event, which broadened out the signifier "Asylum" to bring in the question of asylum-seekers. That widening of the scope of our work also led to "Psychologists against the Nazis," which responded to the real threat of a growth of fascist organizations in the UK by pointing out that electroshock was developed in Mussolini's Italy and that the "mentally ill" were some of the first victims under Hitler in Germany.

Resistance as an abstract moral good could lead us to empty apolitical complaint about what is being done to us, and some of the complaints about the inadequacy of "resistance" draw attention to that problem (Žižek 2008). However, the production of a new signifying chain that links "resistance" to "psychology" and "politics" gives it a new value. Emptiness itself begins to take on a positive aspect against the efforts of psychologists to tell us what we are thinking and feeling. In this way "resistance" could be thought of as an "empty signifier," something that names the site of our struggle against psychology without filling it in again with psychological terms.

CONCLUSIONS

PPR was, for a moment, an "empty signifier," a site of resistance to the discipline of psychology. In its theory and its practice it presented a puzzle to the psychologists about what exactly it was that we wanted, and it also provoked puzzlement among its own members. It was an unstable formation, and necessarily so, and was uncertain about its role as a switching point to connect other existing campaigns or as component of a broader struggle for democratic psychiatry. It was an experiment, and unlike other kinds of experiments in psychology it was designed to deliberately change what it interpreted. Its very existence was a threat to psychology. Now it is an experiment we must repeat.

NOTES

1 Asylum has a good online presence now at www.asylumonline.net.
2 The PPR Newsletters are available as a historical resource at http://www. discourseunit.com/psychology-politics-resistance/.
3 Michel Foucault, "What Is Enlightenment?" (1984). http://foucault.info/ documents/whatIsEnlightenment/foucault.whatIsEnlightenment.en.html. Last accessed 14 May 2012.
4 Immanuel Kant, "An Answer to the Question What Is Enlightenment?" (1784). http://www.marxists.org/reference/subject/ethics/kant/ enlightenment.htm

5

From Subservience to Resistance: Nursing versus Psychiatry

SIMON ADAM

INTRODUCTION

States of domination, Michel Foucault describes, are those instances when a group "succeeds in blocking a field of power relations, immobilizing them and preventing any reversibility of movement" (Rabinow and Rose 2003, 27). Power relations that involve nursing, psychiatry, and pharmacology are the focus of this chapter. The voices of nurses resisting psychiatry have been emerging for some time now, but with a rather cautious crescendo. Nurses organizing against psychiatry, whose recent work modestly appears in the nursing and social sciences literature, emerged out of powerful discourses. As such, these nurses often stand on unstable political ground. These nurses are the trailblazers, the ruptures in the cooperation of nursing with psychiatry. In this chapter, I start with the idea that this political instability arose out of a resistance to powerful ruling discourses, into which nursing consciousness is perpetually hooked in a state of submission. While the very few radical nursing thinkers have begun a counter-narrative, I call attention to some possible reasons why the majority has not joined in. The discourses of pharmacology and psychiatry, as ruling apparatuses, are my critical focus. I examine the state of domination that has enslaved nursing consciousness, and from which a few nurses have been attempting to break.

RADICAL THINKERS IN NURSING

Cheryl van Daalen-Smith (2011b) brings stark phenomenological attention to women's experiences with electroshock. In her study, seven women speak about their experiences as recipients of electro-convulsive therapy. Van Daalen-Smith provides a visceral rendering of the accounts of the women who described shock as having resulted in "damage and devastating loss" (457). These seven women serve as a small sample exemplifying the harmful effects of electro-shock on people, particularly women. Van Daalen-Smith explicates a contradiction in the perceived benefits of electroshock. According to the nurses she interviewed, electroshock provided a positive outcome for the recipients. Concurrently, van Daalen-Smith (2011) examined the nursing literature that covers electroshock. She reports: "Very often, only the pro-ECT arguments are given, only the pro-ECT research is cited, only the pro-ECT perspectives, themes, and ethics are given a voice. Negative accounts of ECT are rarely to be found" (212). She interrogates the literature, suggesting that there is dishonesty in the balance of positive/negative accounts within it. Van Daalen-Smith (2011), through the critique of certain aspects of psychiatry, pulls away a veil of ignorance that has long obfuscated nursing consciousness. Her very inquiry demands that nurses question the ethics of partaking in ECT and mechanically taking up the biases in the ECT nursing literature.

From another critical perspective, Brad Hagen (2007) writes a compelling critique of the Beck Depression Inventory and of the DSM's depression diagnosis criteria in general. He reports on the theoretical and practical problems inherent in this tool and cautions nurses on its limitations, which include numerous cultural, gender, and theoretical biases. In another inquiry, Hagen and colleagues (2008) probe the ethics of accepting gifts from the pharmaceutical industry. They problematize the pharmaceutical sponsorship of nursing and medical education, particularly the education provided by health care institutions. Hagen and colleagues call into question the motivations and interests of the pharmaceutical industry in pro-viding "free" medical education, directing attention to the nursing code of ethics and specifically to the ethical principle of justice. They remind nurses of their duty to "put forward, and advocate for, the interests of all persons in their care ... [Nurses] should promote appropriate and ethical care at the organizational/agency and com-munity levels ... [and] should advocate for fairness and inclusiveness in health resource allocation" (33). I would extend this call to "fair-ness and inclusiveness" to van Daalen-Smith's caution to nurses regarding the ECT literature. I call upon nursing scholars and nurse researchers to examine, as van Daalen-Smith did, the biases in the ECT literature and to respond to these biases. This very response is an example of advocacy for fairness and inclusiveness in health resource allocation, given that the ECT literature is very much a health resource in the nursing academy.

Although the two players discussed here take up a significant nursing role in resisting psychiatry, they are part of a larger resistance structure that has been cutting away at the foundations of psychiatry for decades. Dissident psychologists, social workers, community activists, and psychiatrists construct powerful counter-discourses that have been shaking psychiatry to its base. That resistance to the medical establishment is politically dangerous is not a phenomenon unique to nursing. Take the late Thomas Szasz, for example – a psychiatrist whose antipsychiatry work plays a powerful role in leading the larger movement. Having started as a psychiatrist only to later form perhaps one of the most powerful critiques against twentieth century psychiatry, Szasz faced tremendous professional and political hardships. While bringing to public light the inherent problems with psychiatry, Peter Breggin, another psychiatrist and an important figure to the movement, experienced long-standing collegial reproach, rejection, and legal retaliation. As an example of his rejection of psychiatry, Breggin describes having partaken in the administration of ECT as "the shame of my life" (Burstow, personal communication, 30 August 2012). Whether through the critique of literature, clinical practice, or business relations, nurses too joined this much larger critique of psychiatry. It is noteworthy that a more extensive literature review could not be done, given that such thinkers are a rare occurrence in nursing. This raises a few questions: why is it that a handful of the thousands of nurses have taken this stand? Why is it that despite the obvious ethical violations psychiatry commits, nurses remain silent? What are the institutional conditions under which this silence comes to be? In the following section, I provide possible reasons for this problem in and for nursing.

TWO DISCOURSES AND A NURSE

It is worth fully citing Dorothy Smith's idea of discourse. Dorothy Smith (2005) explicates a discourse as: "Translocal relations coordinating the practices of definite individuals talking, writing, reading, watching, and so forth, in particular local places at particular times. People participate in discourse, and their participation reproduces it. Discourse constrains what they can say or write, and what they say or write reproduces and modifies discourse. Though discourse is regulated in various ways, each moment of discourse in action both reproduces and remakes it" (224). Discourse shapes consciousness, constructs a certain way of knowing phenomena, and to that effect, navigates the actions of those it encapsulates. The various seemingly mundane and taken-for-granted routines, objects, and languages are the powerful elements that hold discourse together and navigate people. They are texts, procedures, and routinized utterances such as "vital signs stable," "patient received alert and oriented," "the patient has a flat affect," and so on. These are the elements of discourse of which Dorothy Smith speaks that mediate the translocal relations that coordinate people's activities. It is important to interrogate these elements, because by their very nature of being routine and seemingly mundane, they implicitly dictate a certain way of knowing for nurses – a specific consciousness from which to practice nursing. It is beyond the scope of this chapter to analyze the major discourses that impact nurses. However, two prominent discourses produce the "mental health" consciousness of the nurse, and these are pharmacology and psychiatry.

THE DISCOURSE OF PHARMACOLOGY

Most of the nurses' medication knowledge is shaped by the discourse of pharmacology. Nurses assimilate their medication knowledge first in the nursing academy. This knowledge becomes concretized on the job by various texts and through various workplace-learning processes, such as orientation programs, in-services, workshops, and drug-sponsored educational sessions. Drug trial literature, medication manuals and reference guides, pocket cards and other such tools, dosage calculation tests, as well as the clinical application of all this information are elements absorbed by nurses from the discourse of pharmacology. For the nursing student and the novice nurse, the action of "tying" the theory together in applying pharmacology knowledge in the clinic is an example of a textually mediated action. This means that a specific text such as a dosage calculation exam authorizes, under the surveillance of a nurse educator, specific knowable things about drugs, their "indication,"

application, and the implications for their use. This textual authori-
zation must also inhibit certain knowledge from being taken up.
This is the work of the translocal relations coordinating through
text – authorizing a certain knowledge yet constraining what nurses
can say, as Dorothy Smith suggests. What the nurses know, in such
a case, is a type of knowledge that has been pre-packaged by the
institution. For example, pharmacology education in acute care
institutions places the nurse in a discourse of efficiency and safety.
In other words, learning about medications and medication administration is only relevant in the context of efficiency and patient
safety (see Dyjur, Rankin, and Lane 2011). Pharmacology also
appears in the form of material imprinted with drug companies'
information, such as pens, paper pads, pocket organizers, lanyards,
buttons, posters, and so on. These too are business strategies that
are in a constant relation with the nurse, and shape his or her consciousness in a specific way. They are cues that consistently stimulate
nurses' sensorium and reinforce that a pharmaceutical response to
psychosocial suffering is indeed the most appropriate response. Such
items, and their creation, occur away from the bedside, in a place
that Dorothy Smith (2005) calls the translocal. In these diverse
ways, the discourse of pharmacology creates a rather accessible
presence for the nurse in a way that is inescapably submerging. Drug
guides, online reference material, workplace learning activities, and
pharmaceutical marketing materials play a dominant role, as major
elements of the discourse of pharmacology, that shape the consciousness of the nurse. In fact, even non-medication related educational
sessions, such as for example training nurses on the use of a new
intravenous catheter, are often sponsored by drug companies that
have an implicit presence. In teaching hospitals, drug trial research
is the thing of today. At any given point, several drug trial studies
may be in progress, whose preliminary findings are progressively
communicated to nurses. This too creates a sort of competitiveness
between drugs as to the "best drug of choice" to treat "mental illness." What this also does is validate where the institution's priorities are: In the progressive "refinement" of drugs.

THE DISCOURSE OF PSYCHIATRY

The work of psychiatry pivots around the DSM. "Mental disorders"
are defined in this text, out of which various psychiatric treatment

modalities and techniques are theorized to "treat" such disorders. The DSM is the starting point in a process that begins with the identification of "illness" and ends with an intervention that may include the medicating, electrocuting, or incarcerating of the "patient." As psychiatry's core text, the cognate disciplines, nursing included, borrow their mental health/illness knowledge from the DSM. The discourse of psychiatry, stemming out of the statistical aggregation of "abnormal" behaviour dubbed mental illness, penetrates the consciousness of nurses and nursing scholars. Psychiatry codifies and categorizes human behaviour in the form of disorders and illnesses, updating them every several years. The DSM, however, does not make an appearance for the nurse in the clinic. Rather, in the form of abbreviated concepts and categories, inserted into the nursing documentation forms, assessment guides, and various legal forms, for example, the Ontario Ministry of Health's Form 1.[1] The Form 1 is the document that authorizes the psychiatric evaluation of the patient, and in the process helps shape the psychiatric assessment. Most of the nurse's work revolves around assessment and documentation tools, which often differ from one department to the next but carry similar elements, which guide the nurse's assessment in a similar way across departments. Very little physical assessment is done on mental health units, where the bulk of the nursing assessment time is taken up by cognitive and behavioural evaluations. The documentation tool guides the work of the nurse to, for example, look for cues or evidence of potential or actual self-harm, document the anxiety level of the patient, note appropriate eye contact, look for insight into illness, and so on. Other discursive elements include educational workshops specifically addressing the care of the "mentally ill," orientation curricula, and historical records of patients' previous hospitalizations.

NURSING ETHICS, BUT SO WHAT?

In contemporary acute care institutions, which are driven by discourses of efficiency and fiscal micromanagement, nurses are often caught in the grind of task-oriented care. Nursing work is constantly monitored, evaluated, and recreated in various ways to respond to direct budgetary cutbacks disguised as ideas of safety, access, and accountability. The consistent emphasis on tasks for the perfect mechanical execution of patient care is what produces the nurse as a drone-like institutional actor often scurrying to do his or her work. It is not unusual that nurses do not get a lunch break or leave their shifts on time, let alone have the time to create any kind of authentic relationship with their patients. That nurses are allowed no time to complete the necessary tasks to render good quality care is an understatement.

Nursing ethics teach us that the nurse ought to act with moral integrity, provide dignity, and support patient autonomy, beneficence, and justice.[2] Ethicists suggest that as nurses, we must respond to the call of our patients, even when we feel that responding so risks compromising our sense of professional and personal integrity (Yeo and Moorhouse 2002). Such principle-based ethics assume that the nurse is first of all aware that an ethical violation is being committed in order to then identify which principle has been breached. Recount the description of the two discourses above and recall the various elements that come into play with the consciousness of the nurse. It is important to note that such elements are only a small example of what perhaps can be an infinite number, all of which make up discourse and its operations. A nurse caught in a minute-to-minute grind of producing institutionally-authorized "efficient" care is strategically navigated by the various translocal relations, such as the nursing assessment form, the assessment itself, its intricate technique, and the method of its documentation. To avoid describing in too mechanical a way how discourse produces the actions of the nurse, I will maintain that discourse is too complex, unstable, and always changing.[3] Moreover, various overlapping discourses make this production of actions and of consciousness even more unstable and difficult. However, mapping out a clinical example may demonstrate how multiple discourses, in this case those of pharmacology and psychiatry, reinforce and reproduce one another in a synergistic fashion, using the nurse as the agent of their reproduction.

A patient is brought into the emergency department by the police. The "presenting complaint" is that the young man was arguing with his mother, the argument became heated, voices became elevated, and he picked up a glass mug and threw it against the wall. The mother became frightened and called the police. Given that the young man has a "history of mental illness," the police arrested him under the Ontario Mental Health Act and brought him to the emergency department for a psychiatric assessment. The receiving nurse greets him in his room, and asks him to undress and wear a hospital gown. His belongings are gathered into a patient belonging bag and immediately removed from the room. An assessment form is initiated by the clerk, stamped with his identifying information, and placed on his chart. The nurse methodically goes through the assessment, completing a quick physical assessment, then a nursing psychiatric evaluation that involves delving into the patient's history of illness, medications, and current state of mental affairs.[4] The assessment quickly proceeds to focus on the presenting issue (violence) and is navigated by cues preprinted in the assessment form to proceed towards explicating triggers, further potential violence, possible involuntary committal, and so on. In the assessment form, the nurse screens for risk, looking for "risk symptoms" such as suicidality and past attempts, self-harming behaviours, and history of violence. A substance use history and a legal history are also obtained and documented, and a mental status exam is completed. Using the data gathered, a pre-diagnosis impression is formulated, and then a psychiatrist provides the diagnosis. While looking for psychocognitive reasons for the cause of the behavioural "problem," the nurse also considers the patient's medications and considers whether or not they are "effective" and whether or not doses need to be increased or new ones should be added. In a few short minutes, the nurse interviews the patient, and works towards understanding, from a pharmaco-psychiatric point of view, the alleged violent event, its potential causes, and possible treatments. The nurse then moves on to formulate a nursing plan of care.

The example above is a routine and common occurrence in the work of the nurse in the emergency department. It would appear that there are no ethical violations taking place during this nurse-patient encounter. The nurse follows a structured relationship-building exercise, provides specific instruction to the patient, completes an appropriate physical and mental health assessment, and works out a plan of care. All this occurs in a fast-paced environment laden with high demands on the time of the nurse. Racing to make care ends meet, the nurse is left with having to complete tasks and with no room to appreciate the patient phenomenologically. During the often-frenzied attempts at a complete "nursing process," which involves an assessment, a plan, interventions, and an evaluation (Wilkinson 2006, cited in Garber O'Brien and Tamlyn 2010), little to no time is left to stand back and reflect. Given that the nurse is consistently entrenched in institutional sequences of speedy mechanical execution of care, how then, can he or she pause to critique any clinical situation? Where is the space in which a nurse is allowed to ethically ponder an incident, reflect, and emerge with a critical understanding of it? Nursing critique does not extend beyond the biomedical paradigm. If it were to do so, the nurse in the example above might take issue with the patient being labeled violent, his being arrested and deemed mentally ill, and with her own practice that stripped the patient of autonomy and dignity. Suddenly, the patient's medications would become problematic; the power relations between the patient and the police, physician, and the nurse would produce ethical discomfort; and the very idea of the patient being mentally ill would become unstable. I turn to some of Michel Foucault's (1977) work to examine why this kind of critique is rare at the bedside.

NO ROOM FOR ETHICS, ONLY DOCILE BODIES

Foucault theorized the idea of the docile body (Foucault 1977a). He suggested that a "mechanics of power" was created, "which defined how one may have a hold over others' bodies, not only so that they may do what one wishes, but so that they may operate as one wishes, with the techniques, the speed and the efficiency that one determines. Thus discipline produces subjected and practiced bodies: 'docile' bodies" (138).

In the contemporary clinic, a similar docility is being produced in nursing. The entrenchment in the ruling discursive operations that Smith (2005) calls the ruling relations is binding for the nurse. The repetitive engagement in such a practice and other routinely executed care processes makes for the "practiced body" of which Foucault speaks. This "practice" is what perfects the institutionally premeditated actions of the nurse – that is, the actions that are coordinated by the discourses of pharmacology and psychiatry.

These practiced bodies are never left alone to "practice" as independent bodies of free social agents. Nurses make up the largest number of caregivers in most health care institutions in Canada, which places them at the centre of most administrative fiscally oriented and efficiency related project reviews. Given that nurses dramatically impact the bottom line of the institution, their work is closely monitored and often harnessed to support many such projects. Nurses, therefore, are well practiced in the art of being governed. Critiquing psychiatry, its practices, its ethics, the labeling of patients, the very practice of nursing itself, therefore, is a distant reality. It is by way of this discursive containment of the docile nurse that most of the nurses have not and do not join radical voices. What then, can nurses do to start an emancipatory counter-narrative, as van Daalen-Smith and Hagen have? I maintain that bedside nurses too, as nursing scholars and researchers do, possess the power to critique, to call into question, and to resist unethical practices. To make suggestions about how this counter-narrative can begin, I turn to a salient concept in nursing that quickly became a buzz-word, and that is the idea of critical thinking.

NURSES AS CRITICAL THINKERS

Three prominent ideas of the concept of critical thinking currently occupy nursing textbooks. The Foundation of Critical Thinking suggests that critical thinking involves employing an art in order to analyze and evaluate thinking with the idea to improve it (Paul and Elder 2006, cited in Garber O'Brien and Tamlyn 2010). Another view of the concept comes from the work of Alfaro-LeFevre (2009), who suggests that critical thinking involves "good problem solving and commitment to look for the best way, based on the most current research and practice findings" (as cited in Garber O'Brien and Tamlyn 2010, 4). The third, and perhaps the most helpful definition, comes from the Canadian Nurses' Association (CNA). The CNA defines critical thinking as: "A complex, active, and purposeful process encompassing the essential skills of interpretation and evaluation and requiring the RN to go beyond the role of performance of skills and interventions" (CNA 2007, as cited in Garber O'Brien and Tamlyn 2010, 4). According to the CNA, critical thinking, "Compels the RN to identify and challenge assumptions, use an organized approach to assessment, check for accuracy and reliability of information, distinguish relevant from irrelevant, normal from abnormal, recognize inconsistencies, cluster related information, identify patterns and missing information and draw valid conclusions based on evidence, identify different concurrent conclusions and underlying causes, set priorities, and evaluate and correct thinking" (ibid). Although the CNA's definition applies to critical thinking in the clinic, I also see nurse educators applying this on a sociopolitical level. It is the same sort of challenging of assumptions that Hagen and van Daalen-Smith did when they stepped outside of the discourses that governed their consciousness. It is the critique that arises out of the space to resist and talk back, for example, to the academic psychiatrist who lodged a complaint against Hagen for teaching out of an anti-psychiatry textbook (B. Hagen, personal communication, 3 July 2012). It is the very critique out of which a humanistic vision for nursing care arises, one that facilitates a platform for the voice of the electro-shocked patient that tells a strikingly different story than what is narrated to nurses by the discourse of psychiatry.

Nurse educators, to begin, must fully appreciate the potential of the power they possess, once they recognize that they too can begin a critique of psychiatry. To mitigate the risk of appearing politically naïve here, let me suggest that beginning such a critique is not without risk. For the nurse clinician, the risks stemming from critiquing psychiatry or psychiatric practices may involve being labeled a pessimist or gaining a reputation for being too critical a practitioner, and often being dismissed by colleagues and nursing leadership. For the nurse academic, the risk can range from one's views simply being dismissed, to difficulty in obtaining access to conduct research, to rejection of potential publications, to dismissal! The radical nursing thinkers did not engage in critique without such risks, as others did long before nursing joined in (e.g. Thomas Szasz and Peter Breggin). However, as Paul and Elder (2006) suggests, critical thinking is the artful analysis and evaluation of thinking with a view to improving it. This art is the strategic way to step outside of ruling structures that authorize what nursing consciousness knows. As radical nurses, psychiatrists, psychologists, social workers, and other activists risked repudiation and suppression, they realized that the areas where they encountered more resistance were the ones they ought to investigative, question, critique, and resist. Under the auspices of academic freedom, nursing scholars, once ready to fully be as critical as the C N A suggests we ought to be, can continue the crescendo of critical voices.

Drawing on our ethical training and from the strength of our personal moral bases, all nurses, scholars, and clinicians alike can resist. Clinicians must interrupt the institutionalized, task-oriented nursing work that has become the thing of contemporary health care institutions and realize that a human-relational nursing approach is possible. Levine states: "Ethical behavior is not the display of one's moral rectitude in times of crisis. It is the day-to-day expression of one's commitment to other persons and the ways in which human beings relate to one another in their daily interactions" (1977, 846). In relating to their patients, nurses can invoke empathy – the capacity to understand another's feelings and provide compassion. Through every interaction in every nurse-patient relationship, nurses can, through empathic critique, resist task-oriented nursing and make space in their consciousness to disrupt this ruling. Clinicians can start by casting doubt on the pathologization of human pain and human behaviour. An instability of the notion of "mental illness" can begin a cascade of changes. Once clinicians and academics together take up the falsity of "mental illness," an alternate consciousness may emerge, one that will break free from the chains of psychiatric ruling.

NOTES

1 "Form 1 – Application by physician for psychiatric assessment," Ministry of Health and Long-Term Care (2000), http://www.forms.ssb.gov.on.ca/mbs/ssb/forms/ssbforms.nsf/FormDetail?openform&ENV=WWE&NO=014-6427-41. Last accessed 3 June 2012.

2 "Code of Ethics for Registered Nurses: Centennial Edition," Canadian Nurses' Association (2008), http://www2.cnaaiic.ca/CNA/documents/pdf/publications/Code_of_Ethics_2008_e.pdf. Last accessed 13 March 2012.

3 Although I make use of Smith's idea of discourse, it is Foucauldian theory on which she draws to carve out this idea of discourse. For more on Foucauldian discourse, see Foucault (1970).

4 The nuances of the processes of patient registration and assessment may differ somewhat between hospitals; however, the processes by which patients are taken through triage assessments, registrations, and nursing and medical assessments are very similar across most acute care institutions in Canada.

6

Developing Partnerships
to Resist Psychiatry
within Academia

PETER BERESFORD AND ROBERT MENZIES

INTRODUCTION

If we are to make better sense of practice and theory in relation to resisting psychiatry in academia, then we will need to gain a better understanding of two recent and related developments. These are: first, the emergence of "service user involvement" in and beyond psychiatry, and second, moves beyond professional, to more inclusive partnership-based and collaborative approaches to opposition to psychiatry. In recent years, there has been an increasing international interest in including the perspectives, comments, and presence of "mental health service users" in both academic and policy settings. This has been framed in different ways in different countries, for example, as "user" or "consumer" involvement, "community engagement," and "empowerment." This is because both nationally and internationally, there is little consensus about language or understandings. There is no agreed-upon language, or conceptualization around user involvement. In the UK, the term most often used is "service user," although some people reject this as passive and unhelpful. Some prefer "psychiatric system survivors," others see this as confrontational and unhelpful. Some service users seek to reclaim the language of "madness"; others see it as inevitably pejorative.

Not only mental health service users, but a wide diversity of groups associated with long-term use of health and social care services have been included as "service users," ranging from older and disabled people, to people with life-limiting and long-term conditions, people living with H I V / A I D S, and people with learning difficulties. Other terms are also used for user or consumer involvement, like partnership, engagement, and participation. In some countries, rather than service user, there is talk of self-help, advocacy, and mutual aid activities and groups, which have a far longer history. Different terms for "service user" emerged as having a different significance at different times, in different countries, and for different stakeholders. "Client," "service consumer," and in some settings, "patient" are all used. In the U S A, for example, advocacy groups tended to favour the term "consumer," while social workers used the word "client." We therefore begin with a problem since we do not have a shared language and what is acceptable for some is demeaning and incomprehensible to others. In this discussion, for simplicity's sake we will use the term mental health service user / survivor, treating it as a political identity that acknowledges the oppression inherent in the existing role, while seeking to be as inclusive as possible semantically (Beresford 2005a). There have been many reasons for this development, but conspicuous internationally, there have been two very different impulses.

THE CONFLICTING ORIGINS OF INVOLVEMENT

The first of these was the political shift, initially framed in terms of the emergence of a "new political right," opposed to state intervention and committed to "free enterprise economics." More recently this has been reframed in terms of neoliberalism, with a powerful commitment to the market, deregulation, reduction in public spending, and a globalised economy. These political and economic developments have both been strongly associated with the rhetoric of consumerism and as pressure has increased for human and public services to be provided by the market, there has been a growing emphasis on the "service user" as an active and involved consumer, contributing to their own well-being both financially and as active agents, as well as being consulted and market researched, like consumers of any other goods or services (Simmons, Powell, and Greener 2009).

The second pressure for participation has come from the emergence of international "service user" movements, most conspicuously the disabled people's movement, but also notably the mental health service user/psychiatric system survivor movement. While these movements have varied, between different countries and between different groups of service users, they have generally been underpinned by a central concern to have more say, to act on their own behalf, and to democratize policy and practice. Generally rights, rather than being welfare based, have developed their own cultures, histories, ideas, theories, struggles, and collective action and have begun to impact on wider policy and thinking (Oliver and Barnes 2012).

As has often been observed, the politics of the supermarket do not necessarily sit comfortably with the politics of liberation. Consumerism and democratization can make uncomfortable bedfellows. This is certainly true for the politics of participation and involvement, where the two competing forces, market-driven neoliberalism and user-led ambitions for empowerment, have encouraged confusion and misunderstanding as to the aims and purpose of user involvement. It is the tensions between these two that explain many of the difficulties and shortcomings increasingly recognized in relation to such user or public involvement.

Involvement based on consumerist consultation is very different from involvement based on a democratic model committed to changing the distribution of power between services, service users, and professionals and increasing service users' say and control. While one is essentially concerned with feeding into dominant professional understandings with the locus of decision-making remaining unchanged, the ambition of the other is to develop different user-led discourses and user knowledge based on direct experience, with the aim of changing where power lies and understandings and responses to the personal and political situation of service users (Beresford 2010).

Not surprisingly, power inequalities between state and citizens, psychiatry and service users, have tended to mean that consumerist understandings of user involvement have predominated over democratizing ones. Thus the dominant model of user involvement has been based on a managerialist/consumerist approach, even though its emergence has provided windows of opportunity for service users and their commitment to democratization. What this has tended to mean, however, is that the involvement of service users internationally has more often been used to feed into and reinforce existing structures, interpretations, and models of policy and professional practice than to challenge these.

DEVELOPING COUNTER DISCOURSES OR BEING SUCKED INTO PSYCHIATRY?

This tendency was highlighted by one of us (Menzies 2010[1]) in an earlier discussion of a petition circulated by the then-president of the Vancouver/Richmond branch of the Schizophrenia Society of British Columbia (Inman 2007) in protest against the 2008 "Madness, Citizenship and Social Justice" conference held at Simon Fraser University (SFU) and concerned with organizing resistance against psychiatry. It is worth looking at this petition more closely within its wider context, and in association with other equivalent examples.

In her criticisms of the human rights conference (which was still in its planning stages at the time), the originator of the petition – one Susan Inman, author of *After Her Brain Broke: Helping My Daughter Recover Her Sanity* (2010) – essentially upheld a psychiatric standpoint. The petition, which was sent to the conference funders and SFU President (among others), was clear in its adherence to "scientific" models that equated emotional and spiritual distress with biogenetically-based brain disease. "The 'medicalization' of serious mental illnesses that you object to," asserted Ms Inman, "has, in fact, dramatically improved the situation of people with mental illnesses and the families who care for them. It has lead (sic) to improved treatments, better research, decreased stigma, and improved public understanding of these devastating brain disorders."

Further, the petition condemned the supposed failure of the event to include the perspectives of psychiatrists and mental health service users' families.[2] In being so apparently sectarian the conference organizers were said to subvert the very causes we claimed to uphold, by choking off "the voices of people whose lives are dedicated to improving the situations of people who live with serious mental illnesses: families and mental health professionals whose work is based on scientifically established best practices" (2007). The document concluded by challenging the very right of the conference to receive governmental funding: "I am surprised," wrote Ms Inman (2007), "that a major university and the major Federal agency promoting research in the humanities and social sciences[3] are comfortable funding a conference that is exploring a major social issue from such a deeply biased perspective."

On first reading, as argued in the earlier paper (Menzies, 2010), it is tempting to brand such antipathy toward human rights initiatives in mental health as "backlash," in the reactive sense of that term. But just as Walby (1993) argues in another context, the "backlash" metaphor is a limited one. In practice we are contending with something far more entrenched and enduring than merely a defensive reaction against gains by anti-psychiatry and psychiatric survivor movements.

In the case of the Schizophrenia Society of Canada (s s c) and its assorted provincial and local branches, we encounter an influential and well-funded advocacy organization which enjoys close ties with the State and corporate sectors. Formerly known as Friends of Schizophrenics, the Schizophrenia Society has been in existence since 1979. The s s c explicitly advances biogenetic understandings of psychosis-as-disease, advocating aggressive forms of psychiatric, pharmaceutical, and legal regulation for people diagnosed with major psychoses. Its members have long supported "early intervention" policies and "assertive treatment" practices in the community. As Erick Fabris has chronicled (2011), the Society's Ontario branch was instrumental in that province's enactment in December 2000 of the infamous Community Treatment Order (c t o) legislation known as Brian's Law. Further, the Society stands for the long-term (and, where applicable, compulsory) use of neuroleptic drugs[4] (not incidentally, a sizable portion of the organization's funding comes from the pharmaceutical companies whose products the Society endorses[5]). At all levels, moreover, the Schizophrenia Society nurtures a close relationship with departments of psychiatry in the country's medical schools. The British Columbia branch, for example, maintains a Medical Advisory Board and has funded the research programs of several psychiatrists and other clinical health professionals on faculty at the University of British Columbia.[6]

Contradictions abound in these cross-cutting relationships. On the one hand, the Society embraces the language of anti-stigmatization, public education and inclusion, "[a]dvocating," according to the home page of its website, "on behalf of individuals and families affected by schizophrenia and in need of mental health help."[7] On the other hand, its intimate ties to medical and corporate elites, coupled with its consistent failure to dialogue with psychiatric survivor and social justice communities, have seriously limited the Schizophrenia Society's breadth of vision while positioning it at the very centre of the policy establishment. In these respects it is no surprise that the Society's leadership would express such enmity toward an event like the SFU conference which was publicly challenging the "science" model of "mental disease" and advancing the autonomy and citizenship rights of psychiatric user-survivors.

Far from being reactive, however, the Schizophrenia Society's ardent promotion of biogenetic psychiatry – like that of its counterparts elsewhere such as NAMI[8] in the United States and SANE[9] in the United Kingdom – is the outgrowth of a systemic, business-as-usual paradigm of control which pervades virtually every aspect of modern life. This paradigm fosters a way of thinking about so-called "sanity and madness," of mental "good and ill health," which follows a long tradition of privileging those who stake their claims to normality and reason on the objectification and exclusion – and too often the persecution – of others. It expresses a deeply ingrained and naturalized way of practicing sanism (Perlin 2003, Poole et al. 2012), of regulating mental "otherness," and of constructing psychiatric "illness" as brain disease.

Yet at the same time there is something new and alarming about the militant brands of latter-day pro-psychiatry activism that animate these organizations. In contrast to prior generations, which witnessed a series of wild pendulum swings between alternative ways of regulating the mind – from the blatant oppressions of somatic psychiatry, eugenics, and Big Pharma, to the "softer" theories and practices of moral treatment, psychoanalysis, and their many variants – in the twenty-first century we are encountering hybrid forms of power over psychiatrized people that are more complex and difficult to engage than ever before.

This "new realist" paradigm for regulating madness – to import a term from criminology (Lea 1987, Matthews and Young 1992) – is fluid, fragmented, reflexive, multi-sited, and therefore able to adjust and reinvent itself constantly. New realist mental health is a moving target. It blurs the boundaries between State and civil society, between the public and private. It blends together the dominant ideas of psy-science (Miller and Rose 2008) and the pharmaceutical empire with popular understandings of sanity and mental "difference." It speaks the language of compassionate care, human rights, populism, inclusiveness, and empowerment. In so doing, it threatens to capture the high ground of liberal rights equality talk. In the deceptive reversal of victim and oppressor that follows suit, it is those activists and academics struggling to carve out spaces for anti-psychiatry and pro-survivor praxis who are the ones deemed to be elitist, exclusionary, unscientific, and outdated.

As we observe in the Schizophrenia Society's response to the above-discussed human rights event at SFU, as well as in main-stream academic and media coverage of similar initiatives elsewhere (see the below discussion of the 2010 PsychOUT conference), to contest the powers of psychiatry is allegedly to undermine the very system of medical ideas and practices on which the lives of 'brain-diseased' people depend. Generations of pseudo-scientific theories, bogus diagnoses, ineffective treatments, invasive interventions and human rights abuses aside, to stand between the psychiatric profes-sional and her/his patient is to place the latter – quite often our very selves – in harm's way. In so doing, if our motives are not downright pathological, they are at least – so the story goes – the product of unreasoning idealism, not to mention naïveté, self-involvement, and ingratitude.[10]

THE GREY ZONE AND THE ACADEMY

In his work on governmentality and the psychological complex, British sociologist Nikolas Rose has written extensively about this new control paradigm and the discourses that sustain it (Miller and Rose 2008, Rose 1999b). Rose's point, following Michel Foucault (1991a), is that the fusion of government and mentality lies at the heart of neoliberalism (see Dean 1999, Gordon 1991). We cannot understand the workings of mental health systems without consider-ing how mind/body control reflects and sustains broader currents of governance – currents that are both remaking our political, eco-nomic, and cultural (and, not incidentally, psychiatric) selves and reworking our relationship to the structures and projects that define our very way of living and being (and of being normal, moral, (re)productive, pacified, self-surveilling, and risk-free).

When it comes to psychiatry and mental "health," the vision advanced by the champions of biogenetic psychiatry and new realist mental health is abidingly neoliberal. The new discourse constructs a psychiatric subject who stands in contrast to the robust, autono-mous, trustworthy, self-governing citizen of the liberal dream. This psychiatrically outcast subject is an alien, an object of sympathy, and/or derision (or simply an object), a victim of a "broken brain" (Andreasen 1985), a being to be spoken and written about (but who cannot take part in the dialogue herself), and above all else "a problem" (Du Bois 2005 [1903]) to be risk-monitored and rehabilitated through the application of law, science, and technology.

Under neoliberalism, and within systems of mental regulation that have prospered under its banner, the psychiatric subject stands outside citizenship altogether. Except as a bundle of traits to be measured and controlled, she who encounters the powers of psychiatry is an invisible, silent (or rather, unheard) outsider, to be domesticated and contained – ill-equipped as she is to take part in this governance project herself. Official "stakeholders" know this to be true, because under neoliberalism the spaces between government, science, mental life, and the body have closed up. Government has, for all intents and purposes, become science, and the science of governance gets applied above all to the minds and bodies of those whose citizenship has been disabled, unmade, literally switched off. Through a quite breathtaking fusion, those of us who happen to think, speak, write, and live outside the neoliberal norms of reason are simultaneously held to account and deemed incapable, unfit, irresponsible, lacking in *mens rea*, in need of "substitute decision-making" – all code words that stand for psychiatric non-citizenship.

And this is where the halls of academia re-enter the conversation. For backing up this new realist mental health system is a vast "assemblage" of technicians of the normal (Foucault 1977a), practitioners of what Rose (1999b) calls the "grey sciences" (administrators, insurers, educators, psychometrists, knowledge workers, assessors, and advisers of all sorts). These technicians work to shore up the neoliberal project by patrolling its boundaries and keeping watch over the countless so-called "deficient," "disordered," and "risky" semi-, non-, and anti-citizens who find themselves shunted to the social margins. For its part, the twenty-first century university has become a key breeding ground for Rose's grey scientists and their involvement in the differentiation, discipline, and exclusion of people deemed psychiatrically unfit for citizenship.

Even so-called "liberal arts" institutions – those which typically lack medical schools or centres of psychiatric training – have become part of this assemblage. In these ways, the modern university has become complicit in establishing the standards by which "normality"

and its absence get defined and measured. Within clinical and forensic psychology programs, criminology departments, health sciences
and studies faculties, and the like, scholars and practitioners who
embrace biogenetic approaches to mental "illness" attract the bulk
of available funding.[11] They are the main gatekeepers for the professional networks and business sponsorships, which pass for
"community-building" in the new corporate academy. They are
front and centre in both media and university (meaning "senior executive") accounts of mental health scholarship. They publish articles
in the highest-ranking journals. And they groom successive generations of students who (with important exceptions) faithfully reproduce their core values and methods. The "grey scientists" (Rose
1999b) who patrol these academic spaces have been successful in
promoting the very kind of objectifying, depoliticizing, reductive,
and essentialist vision of normality and deviance, of health and illness, of sanity and madness that defines the biomedical establishment
within the political and intellectual order of neoliberalism.

THE ALIEN WITHIN US

However, there is an important point to make here. It is not only
policy, services, service providers, professionals, and family members
who may speak from an essentially psychiatric/biological perspective. This is also often true of mental health service users/survivors
themselves/ourselves. That is certainly true from the UK experience
(Beresford 2005b). This is not necessarily because they support it
and give it their allegiance. The likelihood is that this is the only
model of understanding that they have been exposed to. Many mental health service users speak from within an essentially psychiatric
discourse, talking in terms of their diagnosis (often internalizing and
becoming dependent on it), basing their understanding of themselves
and other survivors on individualizing psychiatric interpretations
– because this is all they know. It is often only when mental health
service users begin to get actively involved with others in politicized
survivor organizations and movements, that they have opportunities
to learn about, develop, and share different oppositional ideas. Even
then, not all activists share a common theoretical or philosophical
understanding. Some reject psychiatric conceptualizations; others
are still positioned within it to a greater or lesser extent. What we
may also be seeing in the biomedical rhetoric issuing from some

activist communities (e.g. Inman 2007, 2010) is the internalization of dominant psychiatric understandings. Given the power and legitimacy afforded to these, this is hardly surprising.

When mental health service users were asked about their understanding of models of madness and distress in a UK study, most said that they thought the medical model was unhelpful, and felt that more social understandings were preferable, but participants were heavily divided when asked if they thought that a social model of madness and distress based on the social model of disability would be helpful (Beresford, Nettle, and Perring 2009). The social model of disability, which draws a distinction between individual impairment (the loss or limited function of a limb or sense), and disability (the negative social reaction to people with perceived impairments), has been increasingly influential internationally. At the same time, it has taken a long time for disabled people to become familiar with it and many are still subject to dominant medicalized/biological individual models of disability (Campbell and Oliver 1996, Oliver and Barnes 2012).

WORKING IN PARTNERSHIP TO RESIST PSYCHIATRY

Having begun to explore the complexities and ambiguities of user involvement, we now move to our second focus, moving beyond professional, to more inclusive partnership-based and collaborative approaches to opposition to psychiatry, which involve both service users and professionals. This needs to build on the points raised above: that many service users may still be subordinated to psychiatric understandings, which may have a damaging and divisive effect on the potential for partnership with progressive academics and other professionals. Similarly the latter need to be aware that service users are often and indeed understandably suspicious of them, having some inkling of academic and professional constraints that may operate on them (against service users' interests) and also the competitive and individualizing logic of the academy.

At the same time, these challenges and uncertainties can be turned to advantage. As critical scholars and activists have noted, and often illustrated through practice, neoliberal regimes of governance – the corporate university among them – are self-limiting and primed for resistance along multiple fronts. Throughout the neoliberal world, and on campuses everywhere, openings abound and fault lines penetrate deep. As Dorothy Smith (1990) has written with respect to women and "the conceptual practices of power," these cracks in the foundations of the neoliberal order can be creatively worked to advance the causes of justice, empowerment, and social change. Opportunities for creative partnerships between scholars and activists are arising in all the expected places, as well as many that astonish and inspire. Following bell hooks's (1984) well-travelled metaphor, the margins and centres are forever engaging each other in dynamic and potentially transformative ways.

For reassurance that, pace Yeats, the centre cannot hold and the struggle has never been more vital, we need only look to the remarkable legacy of advocacy that over recent years has issued from the coalition work of academics and grassroots activists; to the arrival of a new generation of critical young scholars, some of whose work is being showcased in this collection; to the global community-building of the International Network Toward Alternatives and Recovery, the World Network of Users and Survivors of Psychiatry, and MindFreedom International's Academic Alliance; and to the "conscientizing" (Freire 1970) initiatives in public education and consciousness-raising about psychiatric rights that are flourishing in all corners of the planet.

In this late modern age, whether we occupy the halls of academia or the corridors of State power or the storefront, office, or street – and whether we are involved in resistance against system oppression or the "life politics" of identity and social position (Giddens 1991) – it is both our burden and our blessing to be endlessly negotiating the intersections between systems of power and the liberating possibilities that these systems reflexively bestow. As with so many other social movements that harbour the potential to change our world for the better, the struggle against (bio)psychiatry – within the academy and beyond – gains its strength from the hard-won ability of people in resistance to penetrate and explode the myth of a seamlessly repressive monolith of mental regulation.

BUILDING OPPOSITION, ALTERNATIVES, PARTNERSHIP, AND INCLUSION IN THE ACADEMY

Crucially, what this demands are new alliances and partnerships between the academy and its professionals and service users and their organizations. As academics committed to challenging the hegemony of psychiatry, and service users committed to freeing ourselves from its damaging dominance, we need to review our relationships. If we are to take these partnerships forward with maximum effectiveness and in equal and inclusive ways, then we must learn new ways of working together and make a long term commitment to such "co-production," as it has come to be called in the UK. Otherwise, as has sometimes been the case, instead of working in true partnership we may find ourselves perpetuating and mirroring the same subordinations, oppressions, and exclusions that operate in the dominant psychiatric and neoliberal systems. The issue is not merely one of reversing "under" and "over" relationships between academics and service users, but of transforming them into more truly equal ones.

While there are still complaints, from service users, of professionals, including radical professionals, still taking the ground from them, rather than ensuring service users opportunities to speak for themselves, there is already much positive experience of partnership and collaboration. Partnerships between academics and service users are already developing internationally, and have the potential to challenge psychiatry in the academy. In the UK, for example, mental health service users/survivors are increasingly being employed in academia to advance user involvement and highlight user perspectives. There are developing examples of high level partnerships, like the SURE (Service User Research Enterprise) project at the Institute of Psychiatry, King's College, London. This is jointly directed by a survivor and non-survivor academic and undertakes large scale user-led research and evaluation projects. The Centre for Citizen Participation at Brunel University, directed by one of us, has a service user advisory group, which includes a large number of mental health service users/survivors who shape its agenda and activities.

Elsewhere we have the example of MindFreedom International's Academic Alliance, which under the directorship of MFI director David Oaks and intern Piers Gooding has, since 2009, been sponsoring a global forum of critical scholars with the goal of integrating the latter into user-survivor activist communities and their knowledge-sharing and social justice projects. What is innovative about this program is that academics are being recruited according to an agenda that is explicitly carved out and directed by activists "in a spirit of mutual exchange"[12] with the realization that "academics who are working to end human rights abuses in the psychiatric system [must] not only be aware of each others' work, but also ... be engaged directly with community-based activists like M F I."[13]

Similar principles are put into practice across assorted other contexts as, increasingly, activists and academics with mental health system experiences and interests find themselves navigating common fields. Conferences like Psycho U T – held in Toronto in 2010, and New York City in 2011 – exemplify the politics of co-production at its best, as scholars in those two cities offered their universities (not without some institutional resistance, and bad press from the local media[14]) as the sites of cross-community engagements and partnerships in the struggle against biogenetic psychiatry. In the U K, the Asylum! events in Manchester have played a similar role in linking critical knowledge production with coalition building and cultural celebration in the transgressively spirited tradition of Mad Pride. The publications that emerge from these and other collaborative ventures – this book, the Canadian Mad Matters collection (LeFrançois, Menzies, and Reaume 2013), and Asylum Magazine being three recent examples – help to raise critical consciousness in important ways. So, too, does the galaxy of user/survivor-oriented, anti-psychiatry, human recovery-focused, and "alternative" mental health advice websites that now populate the World Wide Web.

In the realm of post-secondary education, mad-identified and mad-positive members of university faculties are involved in shaping curricula and mounting courses that aim at correcting the long-standing omission of users' and survivors' words and deeds from conventional academic discourse. In so doing they build on an important and growing legacy of critical teaching and learning that has been pioneered by feminist, queer, anti-racist, and post-colonial scholars, alongside anti-psychiatrists and mad academics working across a broad range of disciplines. Just one among many examples of this trend can be found at Ryerson University in Toronto, where Geoffrey Reaume and David Reville – both self-identified psychiatric survivors and long-time educators, writers, and activists – have been instrumental in crafting an award-winning classroom and on-line course through which, to date, hundreds of students have learned about the history of madness from the standpoint of those who lived it (Church 2013, Reville 2013). Such ventures in political education around mental health criss-cross the boundaries between academy and community in empowering ways. Further, in a context where experiential and critical learning continue to thrive despite the restraints imposed by the neoliberal corporate university, the educators who spearhead these projects can become mentors and role models for students who come to identify themselves as users, consumers, survivors, and/or members of mad communities.

If such trends are to become a routine expression of academic approaches to madness and distress, they will need active, practical support and encouragement. One of the most helpful ways of developing this is to build links – as does MindFreedom International – between academics and their departments and service user/survivor controlled organizations. The latter have a particularly helpful role to play in advancing the practicalities of partnership between professionals and service users as well as supporting service users' empowerment.

Service user trainers equipped with training and qualifications can play a specific part in this, helping service users and academics work better together in inclusive and accessible ways. This can both help progressive academics learn better how to link up with service users and their organizations and also help equip service users with the increased confidence, self-esteem, expectations, and practical knowledge to become equal actors in the endeavour. The official requirement for user involvement in professional social work education courses in England provides a valuable case study of how to take this forward. Since 2003, all professional qualification courses for social work are required actively to involve service users and family carers at all stages and in all their aspects, including for example, student recruitment, assessment and teaching. This has resulted in service users being involved in the selection and assessment of students, in providing teaching, influencing the curriculum, and evaluating courses. Each university department has received ring-fenced/dedicated central government funding to support this and the UK model has become an increasing role model for other professional learning, with major implications for psychology and psychiatry courses (Branfield, Beresford, and Levin 2007; Branfield 2009).

User or survivor controlled research offers a particularly important route to challenging the dominance of psychiatry. It is now emerging as a major new research approach, drawing on feminist, black civil rights, LGBTQ, and community education studies and underpinning a significant and growing number of national and international research projects, employing qualitative, quantitative, and mixed methods. User or survivor controlled research makes it possible to develop a counter discourse to psychiatry, based on survivor knowledge and "lived experience" that is evidence-based and which can challenge the "scientism" of psychiatry, where mental health service users shape the research question and focus, are involved in carrying out the research, producing its findings, disseminating them, and deciding on follow-up action and are in control of all these aspects of the research process. From small starts, this is now emerging as a credible research methodology, with a growing canon of work and rising influence (Sweeney et al. 2009). It is helping to shift the focus from narrow medicalized and individualized interpretations of madness and distress to broader social understandings and responses that take into account the experience and context of mental health service users/survivors, all the while building their own knowledge base.

Not only are specific roles being developed for service users in UK universities, for instance, to advance user involvement. The increasing emphasis on participation is encouraging more people with lived experience as disabled people and mental health service users to become both students and educators and to be "out" about their experiences. However, if this is to develop effectively, it will also need the determined and systematic application of anti-discriminatory policy and practice and for mental health service users, serious revisions in syllabuses that are still influenced by psychiatry, to challenge their inherent "madist" – the equivalent of "disablist" (Oliver and Barnes 2012) – logic, assumptions, and oppressiveness.

It is also likely to be helpful to strengthen links between nascent "mad studies" and burgeoning international disability studies. As well as strengthening their joint understandings and exploring the relations of their theory and modeling, it is important to build connections between mad activism and studies, on the one hand, and disability activism and studies on the other (Campbell and Oliver 1996; Beresford and Campbell 2004). We already have powerful examples from the world of disability activism of how disempowered service users can be supported to be equally involved in the activities of the academy. One such example is supporting people with learning difficulties to carry out their own research, where they receive support, but stay in control (Brennan, Forrest, and Taylor 2012).

CONCLUSIONS

Having said all this, we have to acknowledge that psychiatric models are powerful. They are heavily ingrained in public, political, and academic consciousness. The job of challenging them will be a demanding, difficult, and long term one. In the ways that we have canvassed in this chapter, the road ahead is all the more daunting for the presence of twenty-first century forms of governance that have sponsored a toxic blend of neoliberalism and biogenetic psychiatry in the mental health system and the many institutions and communities (including the academy) with which the mental health system intersects. The impact of these regimes cannot be overstated. Nor can the pace and intensity with which they have transformed all our lives.

Just as biopsychiatry constructs us as the inert and inept objects of scientific and chemical technology, so neoliberalism tries to isolate us from each other with the message that we are responsible solely for maximizing our own usefulness as economic beings, managing our risk to ourselves and others, and generally falling into line with the reigning order of things. Even within post-secondary centres of teaching and learning – among the key custodians, in our world, of critical thinking and engagement – these twin pillars of science and governance have colluded to promote the medical model of mental "illness" and complicate efforts to challenge the psychiatric status quo.

Yet as we have also witnessed above, and as this book of essays passionately attests, this sword, too, cuts both ways. From grassroots community activism to global democracy movements, the neoliberal age has also been a time of unprecedented human rights awareness, advocacy, and coalition building (Chomsky 2012). When it comes to mental health, psychiatric survivors, system users, and mad pride activists have been the vanguard of a collective movement (however partially formed and loosely coupled) that has the potential, in David Oaks' words (2008), to launch a genuine "nonviolent revolution." This is not to say that biomedicine and neoliberalism will not continue to colour our experiences of emotional and spiritual diversity and distress, nor that many of us will not still internalize the values and beliefs these systems promote. Nor, for that matter, can we discount the contradictions that underpin, and sometimes undermine, various strands of our communities (Diamond 2013). Yet through the many solidarity projects, partnerships, and experiments in empowerment and inclusion that are flourishing worldwide – and through the alliances that we are forging with kindred movements from disability rights to post-colonialism to queer and trans emancipation – the dialectics of oppression, resistance, and social change will continue to play out (as ever, in unforeseeable ways) as the future unfolds.

New discourses are being developed by mental health service users/survivors out of their situation and the present neoliberal politics and economics. While these are constantly at risk of being overshadowed and overpowered by psychiatry in association with the dominant politics, nonetheless they represent a fundamental break from both. We can have no idea what impact this new development will ultimately have, because it is essentially unprecedented. It is resulting in changes within people and beyond in their social, cultural, and political worlds, as a result of their collective action. Such new discourses offer routes to and the promise of both bottom-up and top-down change. But while we cannot know what future it has, it is difficult to believe other than it is the star that the academy and its professionals must hitch themselves to, if they are to be true to their responsibilities to pursue knowledge, rigour, social justice, and the rights and interests of the world in which they exist. They have a key role to play here in partnership, but equally an opportunity to fulfil their true academic ethos.

NOTES

1 R. Menzies, "Navigating the Grey Zone: Advocacy for Psychiatric Citizenship in the Academy" (paper presented at the Psycho UT Conference, Toronto, 7–8 May 2010), http://individual.utoronto.ca/psychout/panels/menzies.html. Last accessed 7 September 2012.

2 In fact, the conference organizers extended an open invitation to participate, and no paper or panel submissions were rejected. Several psychiatrists and other clinicians spoke at the conference, and numerous delegates had family members with histories of involvement with the mental health system.

3 The Social Sciences and Humanities Research Council of Canada was one of the conference funders.

4 See the s s c's "Position Paper: Early Intervention in Schizophrenia," available at http://www.schizophrenia.ca/docs/EarlyInterventionIn Schizophrenia.pdf.

5 Among its most generous supporters, the 2012–13 Report of the Society's Ontario chapter lists Lundbeck Canada Inc., Bristol-Myers Squibb Canada, Pfizer Canada, Hoffman-La Roche Limited, Sunovion Pharmaceuticals Canada Inc., Novartis Pharmaceuticals Canada Inc., Pfizer Canada Inc., and Janssen Inc.

6 The b c chapter's Research page includes sections entitled "More Clues in the Genetics of Schizophrenia," "New Antipsychotic Review: z e l d o x," "Twins Help Find Cause of Schizophrenia," and "The Insanity Virus" (the latter item favourably cites a 2011 article in *Discover Magazine* with the caption: "Schizophrenia may not be just a matter of bad genes or bad luck. A growing group of psychiatrists says the real culprit is a virus entwined in every person's d n a." See http://www.bcss.org/category/ aboutbcss/research/).

7 See http://www.schizophrenia.ca/advocacy_papers.php

8 Founded in 1979 and based in Arlington, Virginia, the National Alliance on Mental Illness (n a m i) describes itself as "the most formidable grassroots mental health advocacy organization in the country." The n a m i website can be found at http://www.nami.org/.

9 s a n e is a mental health charity founded by journalist and campaigner Marjorie Wallace c b e that came to prominence at the time of the tragic killing of Jonathan Zito by the mental health service user Christopher Clunis in 1992. While it is now presented as an organization committed to increasing support and understanding for mental health service users, it came to prominence on an unsubstantiated wave of political and media concern about the increasing risk and danger posed by mental health service users following de-institutionalizing mental health policies in the 1990s (Szmukler 2000; Taylor and Gunn 1999). In fact a major problem facing service users like Christopher Clunis was the lack of available psychiatric help when they sought it.

10 The dominant paradigm of mainstream biogenetic psychiatry is so pervasive that it extends far beyond the clinical professions, pro-psychiatry interest groups, and the general public. As Reaume (2000) has shown in his review of academic portraits of people with psychiatric diagnoses, scholars who profess critical leanings, as well as members of the Left more widely, are by no means exempt from such attitudes. Shortly after the above-mentioned discussion of the Schizophrenia Society petition

appeared in the online proceedings of the Psycho UT conference (Menzies, 2010), one of us [RM] received an email from a sociologist colleague from another university who – citing the case of a young woman whose medications "rescued [her] from bizarre asocial behaviour" and "enabled [her] to function and enjoy life" – characterized my critique of biogenetic psychiatry under neoliberalism as "very misdirected," and declared that my "preferred discourse ... exceeds its own limits," is "absurd (and hurtful) and "appl[ied] ... in an indiscriminate manner." The colleague concluded by advising me: "take off your own ideological lenses and look at the facts of the individual case."

11 For instance, a search of the Canadian Institutes of Health Research (CIHR) data base, using the key words "mental health," shows that the vast majority of the 842 currently funded projects in this field (with grants totalling nearly $150 million) are proceeding from an explicitly clinical and/or biogenetic perspective. Research which embraces explicitly user-survivor, critical and/or feminist approaches to the study of psychiatry and mental health is conspicuously absent from this list.

12 "MindFreedom Academic Alliance: MindFreedom's Network of Allies in the Academic World," D. Oaks (2012). http://www.mindfreedom.org/campaign/development/academic-alliance-launch. Last accessed September 7, 2012.

13 See Gooding in: "MindFreedom Academic Alliance: MindFreedom's Network of Allies in the Academic World."

14 See, for example, Joseph Brean's article on the first Psycho UT conference in Toronto, which characterized the meeting's delegates as a "motley bunch" of ideologues and extremists who were pushing an irrational anti-psychiatry agenda. Joseph Brean. "Mind control." *National Post*, 8 May 2010, 8. For a response to Brean's polemic, see David Oaks' posting on the MindFreedom website: http://www.mindfreedom.org/campaign/media/mental-health-bias/joseph-brean

7

"We Do Not Want to Be Split Up from Our Family": Group Home Tenants Amidst Land Use Conflict[1]

CHAVA FINKLER

INTRODUCTION

There exists a significant scholarly literature that examines psychiatric survivor[2] housing experiences of homelessness (Shartal et al. 2006) as tenants in public housing (Jones et al. 2003) and in supportive housing (Schneider and McDonald 2008). However, there has been little written about psychiatric survivors' experiences living in group homes or boarding homes (Capponi 1992) and, in particular, about how land use law constructs tenants' relationships with one another. This chapter examines the ways in which group home tenants resisted the imposition of medico-legal interpretations of their relationships with one another and subverted definitions of group homes in land use law. Simultaneously, this chapter demonstrates the flexibility and relevance of a psychiatric survivor analysis[3] to scholarly endeavour.

A psychiatric survivor analysis considers the impact of social and legal processes upon psychiatric survivors as central, rather than peripheral, to scholarly understanding. Such an analysis directly challenges conventional social and legal practice (Finkler 2013). Although many survivors offer a psychiatric survivor analysis (Beresford 2005b), one need not be a survivor to do so (Kaiser 2001). A psychiatric survivor analysis integrates an understanding of sanism, a form of systemic discrimination that targets psychiatric survivors. There is cumulative evidence of sanism's pervasive presence in multiple milieux. Psychiatric survivors have often had limited access to mental health care (Steele, Glazier, and Lin 2006) and physical health care (Campbell et al. 2007). Psychiatric survivor labourers worked long hours in sheltered workshops or hospitals for little or no remuneration (Reaume 2000). Some survivors were sterilized against their will (Cairney 1996). Until 1988, psychiatric inpatients in Canada did not even have the right to vote in federal elections.[4]

A psychiatric survivor analysis is not a description of psychiatric survivor perspectives or preferences. Rather, a psychiatric survivor analysis examines socio-legal circumstances in the context of sanist power relations. Sanism intersects with other forms of oppression such as ableism (Bahm and Forchuk 2008), adultism (LeFrançois 2011), ageism (Ontario Human Rights Commission 2012), anti-Semitism (Strous 2009), classism (Cran and Jerome 2008), colonialism (Fanon 1968), heterosexism (Daley, Costa, and Ross 2012), racism (Dhand 2011), and sexism (Burstow 2006a). If psychiatric survivors belong to another oppressed group, the discrimination they experience increases exponentially (Ontario Human Rights Commission 2012).

I introduce the concept of a psychiatric survivor analysis as an activist antidote to mainstream land use planning practices, such as zoning, which often ignore psychiatric survivor realities. While policymakers concur that survivor perspectives must be considered when contemplating service provision, the legislature rarely applies a psychiatric survivor analysis to land use law. Similarly, psychiatric survivor analyses are virtually absent from the scholarly planning literature.

Academic articles have been written about psychiatric survivor housing preferences (Forchuk et al. 2006). Researchers could argue that survivors participate in housing studies by offering feedback and, sometimes, by interviewing other survivors (Reeve et al. 2002). However, survivor participation in research is significantly different from psychiatric survivor directed or controlled research (Beresford 2002).

Some academics may support psychiatric survivor housing but nonetheless use offensive language. For example, scholars have referred to psychiatric survivors using phrases such as "service dependent populations" (DeVerteuil 2011; Dear and Wolch 1987).

The term "service dependent populations" suggests that psychiatric survivors engage solely in relationships of dependence. However, psychiatric survivors may participate in reciprocal relationships, sometimes bonding with other survivors.

Survivors on social assistance often do depend on mental health services for their well-being. However, wealthy non-survivors may be equally "dependent" on nannies, housecleaners, and personal trainers. Members of privileged classes pay for services whereas persons living in poverty receive mental health services for free, whether they want them or not. Language that emphasizes dependence as a prominent psychiatric survivor trait reflects an outlook based on the privilege of able-bodiedness and wealth. Two economically divergent groups "depend" on service providers but only persons living in poverty are characterized by relationships of dependence. The latter relationship is marginalized while the former is normalized.

Michel Foucault (1995) portrays the norm as part of a complex system of social control that strictly enforces socially accepted standards of human behaviour, noting: "It is easy to understand how the power of the norm functions within a system of formal equality, since within a homogeneity that is the rule, the norm introduces, as a useful imperative and as a result of measurement, all the shading of individual differences" (184). In response to this intricate web of control, Foucault anticipated resistance. In his essay, *The Subject and the Power*, Foucault maintained: "If it is true that, at the heart of power relations and as a permanent condition of their existence, there is an insubordination and a certain essential obstinacy on the part of the principles of freedom, then there is no relationship of power without the means of escape or possible flight" (Rabinow and Rose 2003, 142). It is precisely the effort to challenge the nature of the "normal" that I wish to describe. In fact, "normal" is not "natural" at all. Rather, in the group home context, the concept reinforces socially constituted differences embedded within planning legislation.

THE ORIGINS OF THE GROUP HOME

While group homes are considered a modern social innovation, they may also have represented one possibility on a continuum of housing options for psychiatric survivors as early as the 1890s in Ontario.[5] Over a hundred years ago, asylum administrators advocated the use of cottages (sometimes referred to as the "villa system") as a means by which to provide greater liberty to inmates within asylum walls. These small homes provided a residential alternative to overcrowded wards in the main hospital buildings.

Today, remnants of the cottage system remain in use in places like Riverview Psychiatric Hospital in Coquitlam, British Columbia (Figure 7.1). Although Riverview Hospital closed in 2012, cottages on the hospital site still house psychiatric survivors in the forensic system. Cottages appear to have been precursors to the modern day group home. They dispersed psychiatric survivor inhabitants within a contained space, permitting "freedom" while retaining control.

Advertisements seeking group home staff appeared in the classified section of the *Toronto Star* as early as 1961.[6] A *Toronto Star* reporter first mentioned group homes in 1963 as an alternative to foster homes for youth (Bruner 1963). Today, social service organizations establish group homes for psychiatric survivors and other marginalized groups.

GROUP HOMES' LEGAL STATUS IN ONTARIO, CANADA

Tensions, both ideological and practical, surround group homes' status in residential areas. The specificity of the group home designation presents an inconsistency. On one hand, the appellation describes a "home," i.e. a residential use. However, provincial government funding in concert with strict municipal regulation is typically associated with institutional settings. Because of this inconsistency, adjudicators have often been asked to determine whether a group home is a home or an institution. Definitions of the group home exist within both provincial statute and municipal bylaws. Usually, definitions of the latter are based on the former.

In Ontario, Canada, s 163 (3) of the Municipal Act contains the governing definition: "'group home' means a residence licensed or funded under a federal or provincial statute for the accommodation of three to 10 persons, exclusive of staff, living under supervision in a single housekeeping unit and who, by reason of their emotional, mental, social, or physical condition or legal status, require a group living arrangement for their wellbeing." The Municipal Act indicates that inhabitants live in group homes due to an impairment. The definition identifies housing for psychiatric survivors as housing for persons with a specific condition, who are not "normal," whose bodies

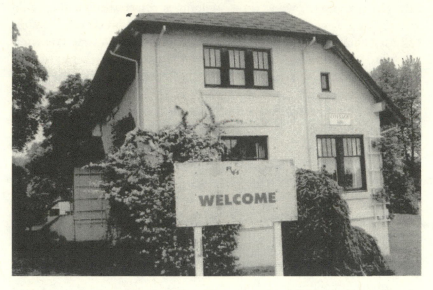

Figure 7.1   An Example of a "cottage" at Riverview Hospital in BC. (Photo by
Chava Finkler, courtesy of Chava Finkler)

and minds do not comply with standards set by legislators and regu-
lators of social behaviour.

Disability studies theorist Rosemarie Garland-Thomson (1997)
wrote, "The term "normate" usefully designates the social figure
through which people can represent themselves as definitive human
beings. Normate, then, is the constructed identity of those who, by
way of the bodily configurations and cultural capital they assume,
can step into a position of authority and wield the power it grants
them" (8). In this theoretical context, group homes are housing created for the "not-normal," not-powerful, not-useful, the social detri-
tus that must be socially deterred. Since psychiatric survivors are the
designated "not-normal," relationships they have with each other
can be considered of only minimal significance. It is precisely because
of this "not normal" status that many mental health professionals
emphasize community integration. In this paradigmatic paradox,
relations between the normal and not-normal are judged to be of
greater import even though the normal are reluctant to relate to
their "not-normal" neighbours.

Amendments to the Municipal Act changed the definition of group
home, deleted the previous phrase "live as a family" and instead,

inserted the term, "single housekeeping unit." Although *R. v. Bell* stipulated that municipalities could zone only the land use (but not the user), group home legislation still describes types of tenants and their relationships with each other. While provincial legislation provides an overriding definition, municipalities exert control by altering the meaning of group home in zoning bylaws. For example, some towns have limited group homes to a maximum of three inhabitants.[7] Other municipalities may enact minimum separation distance requirements that limit the proximity within which group homes can be located (Finkler and Grant 2011).

As Foucault (1995) noted, power is dispersed and exercised in the minutiae of everyday interaction. It is not only cataclysmic events that shape and determine social position but rather the details of daily life that govern subject populations. While provincial statutes govern planning processes in Ontario, zoning bylaws enacted by municipalities have an immediate and daily impact upon citizens. They function as the asylum walls of yesteryear to contain and constrain psychiatric survivor lives.

LAND USE LAW PROCESSES

When organizations wish to establish a group home, they typically negotiate with municipal planners to determine location, structure, number of rooms, etc. Depending on zoning bylaws, a group home may or may not be permitted in the desired area. On occasion, an agency or operator is required to apply for a variance that permits the group home despite a restrictive bylaw. For example, a group home may require a wheelchair ramp that would decrease distance between the house and street. In many circumstances, an inch or two would be insignificant. Property owners receive routine approval for many variances from municipal Committees of Adjustment. However, if neighbours oppose a group home in principle, they can use the requirement for a variance to deny the organization its request.

The sponsoring agency or operator could, in that situation, reconfigure the group home structure or move it elsewhere. If the request for a variance is denied by a municipality, or alternatively, if neighbours wish to challenge group home approval, either side may be able to appeal to the Ontario Municipal Board (OMB), a provincial administrative tribunal. Usually, OMB adjudicators are final arbiters of land use disputes.

CASE STUDY

This chapter is based upon mixed methods research undertaken from 2005–08. Using grounded theory (Glaser and Strauss 1967), I read, analyzed, and coded over 1,000 pages comprised of two OMB case files, thirty-one OMB decisions, a compilation of forty-five municipal bylaws, and transcripts from twenty-six semi-structured interviews. Analyzing the data I identified key themes, including "group home as home, group home as institution." Although this research is part of a larger study investigating the way that notions of disability are socially and legally produced in Ontario planning processes, here I focus on ways in which land use law constructed the group home as a home outside the norm, and the ways in which psychiatric survivor tenants resisted this designation. Municipal minutiae such as zoning bylaws exerted social control. In response, psychiatric survivor tenants resisted socially sanctioned sanism by physically and metaphorically traversing "home" territory.

Scholars identify over-regulation and/or rejection of group homes as manifestations of the Not-In-My-Back-Yard (NIMBY) phenomenon. Instead, I suggest that NIMBY is but one example of sanism in the housing context. As Perlin noted, "The concentrated efforts to 'zone out' group homes and congregate residences for the mentally disabled offers a paradigm of sanist behaviour" (1991, 92).

My case study involved a land use dispute in a mid-sized Ontario town I call Placeville. A private operator wished to open a licensed group home in a pre-existing building, partially located on a flood plain. Prior inhabitants were sixteen members of an extended family. The operator wished to house sixteen tenants, psychiatric survivors who had lived together previously. The operator did not request structural alterations. At the time, Placeville had no group home bylaw. The local Conservation Authority would not approve the group home because its flood plain location could have jeopardized efficient emergency evacuation of tenants.[8]

Flood plain management required that municipal officials contact police and implement local evacuation plans. In an emergency, it was considered more difficult to manage an evacuation if residents had mobility impairments (Conservation Authority Employee). The dangers facing disabled persons in flood situations have been well documented, particularly after Hurricane Katrina (National Council on Disability 2006). In Placeville, pre-existing residential uses were permitted to remain on the flood plain area. However, new residential development was not allowed (Conservation Authority Employee). In the OMB case, the flood plain area covered only a small portion of the group home's back yard. The parking lot, main entrance, and fire escape were all at street level, well above the flood plain. Tenants were psychiatric survivors capable of escaping the premises independently.

Correspondence between the Town of Placeville and the Conservation Authority revealed that the town had no definition of "group home." The planning director nonetheless treated group homes as a residential use. S/he wrote, "The Town while acknowledging a difference between types of group homes and institutional forms of residential care facilities, is evaluating the current application as a group home (as defined by the Town's current Official Plan) as residential use and not as institutional." Planner #1, employed by the Conservation Authority, wrote to Placeville colleagues: "The proposed group home residents will require 24-hour supervision and would appear to fall within the broad institutional intent of the policy ... staff cannot recommend that the proposed use be located in the flood plain since regional storm events are difficult enough for individuals without handicaps to deal with." This comment presumed that tenants had mobility impairments. They did not. The planner also presumed psychiatric survivors required "supervision," a common sanist presumption I noted elsewhere (Finkler 2006).

In a divergent view, the group home operator described flood plain location as a red herring, stating: "There are no people in wheelchairs living in the house. The tenants can run out easily. The last flood in the region was 50 years ago. That's what I went through. Everything they could put in my way, they did." In his/her comments, the operator referred obliquely to prevailing NIMBY sentiment. Neighbourhood opponents stated clearly in interviews that they did not wish to have another group home close to downtown.

In contrast to planners, municipal officials, and the landlord, tenants indicated that they wished to live together because they considered one another "family." Some tenants knew each other from previous homes. One town councillor, present at both the public meeting and the OMB hearing, described a tenant's testimony thus: "One [tenant] spoke beautifully. Some [tenants] have been in the [same] group home for ... close to fifteen years, so they were definitely a family and had not caused any issues within the community in their tenure together … [s/he] touched my soul … [s/he] did not want to be split up from [his/her] family … the only environment [s/he'd] really known." This perspective, describing tenant relationships, is rarely considered in land use deliberations. Usually, the building's presence is negotiated before space is rented. Here, tenants moved together to the new location because they were displaced by fire. The operator may have introduced tenant testimony at the OMB to bolster his/her claims. Nevertheless, tenants prioritized their relationships to one another rather than their relationship to the operator.

By speaking of each other as "family," tenants' testimony resonated with a description written by psychiatric survivor Pat Capponi (1992), who noted in her autobiography, *Upstairs in the Crazy House*, "Imagine being told … for years that you have to be locked up. Then, some clown is standing there, talking about how it's time for you to go; being in hospital for so long isn't good for you. Here's a ticket and an address; a welfare worker will be by to see you, good luck. Imagine you have no more control over this than anything else in your life. This hospital, this staff, the patients, and people you've been locked up with for years have become closer than siblings you no longer remember, but no one seems to mind that for the second time, you've been surgically removed from your family" (29). During deinstitutionalization, the emphasis was on physical placement in the "community." The implications of emotional dis-placement were not considered.

Restrictive forms of zoning not only restricted psychiatric survivor housing, they simultaneously "disciplined" (Foucault 1995) survivor tenants by demanding self-imposed invisibility. This territorial negotiation was evident in the visual relationship between survivor tenants and non-survivor homeowners next door. The operator landscaped the backyard so tenants could congregate there. Tall trees graced each side of the yard, blocking sightlines, and thereby ensuring that tenants remained invisible to neighbours. Tenants, however, refused to adhere to this attempt at visual buffering. Tenants first resisted NIMBY sentiment by testifying at the OMB and then resisted that sentiment again in their own home.

Instead of remaining in the backyard, tenants stood at the front of their premises where they could both see neighbours and be seen by them. Tenants occupied "transitional spaces" (Knowles 2000) such as the parking lot and fire escape, usurping them for their own purposes such as smoking, chatting, or reading the paper. Rather than moving through these areas on their way somewhere else, psychiatric survivor tenants staked their claims to these unmarked territories. Significantly, tenants moved in groups of two or three, rather than as individuals. Their collective identity may have influenced this spatial configuration.

We can understand these spatial negotiations by incorporating Foucault's depiction of the clinical (or observing) gaze. Foucault stated: "The observing gaze refrains from intervening: it is silent and gestureless. Observation leaves things as they are; there is nothing hidden to it in what is given. The correlative of observation is never the invisible, but always the immediately visible, once one has removed the obstacles erected to reason by theories and to the senses by the imagination. In the clinician's catalogue, the purity of the gaze is bound up with a certain silence that enables him to listen" (2007, 131). This all-knowing, medical/visual interrogation, described by Foucault as the clinical gaze, manifested itself in the tensions between psychiatric survivor tenants and their neighbours during the land use dispute. While the clinical gaze often exercises its authority when the powerful examine the weak, in this case study, neighbours in power prevented psychiatric survivor tenants from viewing them. Visual buffering asserted homeowner supremacy since structural changes, such as the transplanting of fully-grown trees and the installation of double trellises blocked sightlines. These moves revealed neighbours' efforts to visually repel the psychiatric survivor gaze while simultaneously insisting tenants be properly "supervised." Negotiations involving visual accessibility reflected power relations between psychiatric survivor tenants and non-disabled homeowners and demonstrated ways in which the landscaped environment can spatially reproduce relations of power and privilege.

ASSERTION OF PSYCHIATRIC SURVIVOR TENANTS AS "FAMILY"

Neither neighbourhood opponents nor Placeville employees challenged tenants' versions of their relationships with each other. It appears that persons related by shared histories of confinement or psychological condition do not fall within definitions of "family" established by nondisabled society. Tenants' assertions to the contrary, therefore, could easily be ignored. Clearly, psychiatric survivors can constitute "family" for one another. The reluctance to view bonds between psychiatric survivors as central, rather than peripheral, exemplifies sanist sentiments.

Tenants' relationship to one another was central to an analysis of the group home. If tenants were "family," the group home was considered a "home." If tenants were not family, the group home was considered an institution. If the group home was a home, it could locate on a flood plain. If the group home was an institution, it could not locate on a flood plain. If the group home could not locate on a flood plain, then the operator would have had to close the group home. Tenants would have been forced to move and be separated from one another. Ultimately, the issue was decided by the O M B. The adjudicator declared: "The Board does not agree that a group home is an institutional use. It is a residence, a "home," for certain persons who qualify to be residents of the group home. It is not a hospital and the residents are not physically sick and therefore incapable of leaving the home in the unlikely event of a regional storm occurring. It is merely steps to the street which is not in the floodplain."[9] The operator subsequently opened the group home and Placeville enacted a group home bylaw.

The tenants in the case study are certainly not alone in their self-identification as "family." In the land use context, Heslin et al. (2011) described sober living homes in which tenants consciously referred to one another as family members. Heslin et al. also referred to a US case in which developmentally disabled persons living in a group home were considered an "alternative family" and noted: "These cases illustrate how public policies and the rhetorically potent concept of family can help validate the close personal relationships of disabled people" (2011, 478). When group home tenants defined themselves as "family," they stressed the importance of their relationships with one another. Tenants were unlikely to choose their roommates (Schneider 2010); these decisions were typically made by staff. Nonetheless, tenants asserted a bond with those who shared their living space. This was no small feat, given the "self-stigma" (Corrigan and Watson 2002) many psychiatric survivors felt.

Self-stigma, or what can be referred to as "internalized sanism," can occur when psychiatric survivors adopt the same values and perceptions non-survivors use to oppress them (Corrigan and Watson 2002). As psychiatric survivor advocate, Judi Chamberlin, wrote in her classic call for survivor autonomy, *On Our Own*: "Like racism and sexism, mentalism infects its victims with the belief in their own inferiority, which must be consciously rooted out. By working together in self-help organizations, ex-patients can gain experience in helping themselves and one another. But the belief in one's own inferiority can continue unless active efforts are made to combat it" (173).

There are good reasons for the creation of a "chosen family."[10] Tenants may develop bonds in order to respond to the challenges inherent in congregate living. Group home situations are often far from ideal. There are tales of abuse[11] and even death (Canadian Medical Association Journal 2002). According to one government policy analyst, inspection and ongoing scrutiny of group homes is crucial: "There have been difficult situations of tenant exploitation. Once, we had only sixty days to locate new homes for a large group of tenants. Now we insist a transfer agency be involved to monitor group homes."

Despite media coverage detailing sometimes intolerable conditions in group homes, evidence in the case study O M B file indicated the operator advocated effectively on behalf of tenants. When the operator examined tenants at the O M B hearing, s/he framed questions in terms of "rights" and asked tenants whether they ought to be able to live wherever they wished. This rights-based approach suggests entitlement to a home, a position uncharacteristic of landlords generally.

Tenants may consider one another family, given the significant periods of time they spend with one another. Problems with public transportation (Muir et al. 2010), lack of access to a vehicle (due to poverty) (Filion 2000), or an inability to drive (due to an impairment)[12] may limit physical mobility outside the home (Gold 2008). In addition, the cost of socializing outside the home can be prohibitive (Miflin and Wilton 2005). Housemates are physically accessible and there is no financial cost associated with social interaction. Furthermore, service providers often "cream" potential tenants (Schneider 2010) offering housing to those most likely to succeed. Therefore it is possible that tenants will be at a similar stage of recovery. Consequently, there may be a built-in degree of interpersonal compatibility.

Some tenants may prefer congregate living as a form of social support. Studies have shown that, for psychiatric survivors, living independently is associated with increased social isolation (Beal et al. 2005). Physical integration in a neighbourhood does not often constitute social integration with local inhabitants (Abdallah et al. 2009). Non-survivor neighbours often reject psychiatric survivor tenants via legal or architectural choices. Neighbours routinely oppose group home presence[13] and if unsuccessful in barring the home, may harass new arrivals[14] or install visual buffering such as frosted windows (Finkler 2006) to block sightlines between properties. Prospective neighbours do not wish to see psychiatric survivors; they also do not wish to be seen by them.

Given frequent rejection by neighbours, group home inhabitants do well to seek support from one another. Certainly, when being deinstitutionalized: "Being relocated together means individuals have ... contacts who may provide support as new relationships are negotiated. Experiences of mental illness and ... a shared history of services often mean that people with mental illness living in the community feel more comfortable socializing with their peers than [they do with] people without the experience" (Forrester-Jones et al. 2012, 11).

Harley et al. noted that "[o]f 79 [research] participants with friends, 75 named someone amongst fellow service users, who they met at hospitals or day centres. They appreciate shared experiences and mutual support" (2012, 1298). Tenants in supportive housing explained they chose other survivors as friends because: "Mental illness can be so isolating that ... many of us are very lonely ... we get socially awkward ... Sometimes, if you share your own wounds it makes it easier for all of us. There are times where it's really helped" (Bendell et al. 2010, 33). Another psychiatric survivor elaborated: "I am more comfortable with people who have had experiences of mental health problems because you do share something and have something to talk about. I haven't been in society for many years .... I can't hold conversations with normal people ... I [would] sooner not be bothered" (Harley et al. 2012, 1296).

Some scholars mention the crucial role reciprocity plays in friendship. Researchers noted: "Participants with psychiatric disabilities who were given monthly stipends, but not matched with a peer with whom to spend the money, tended to use stipends to purchase items for persons who provided assistance in the past" (Wong et al. 2009, 62–3). When considering the centrality of "give and take," perhaps psychiatric survivor tenants felt most comfortable with one another as they could participate in similar forms of reciprocal engagement, i.e. offer emotional support as opposed to financial support. This interplay acknowledges not just common psychiatric history but similar class status.

Tenants' characterization of themselves as a "family" may also have been an attempt to normalize their relationships, i.e. to present themselves, and possibly staff and landlord, as being related to one another. However, this depiction carries with it an uncritical assessment of power dynamics both between tenant and landlord and amongst tenants themselves. Fenby (1991) asserts that defining tenants of a community based residence as a family in fact re-segregates psychiatric survivors, and reinforces patriarchal relationships between tenants and staff: "From the denial of adult sexuality through the use of double bedrooms to the potential for staff to define any deviant behaviour as mental illness, the community residence is a powerful strategy for the social control of disabled people. By keeping clients in one place and under surveillance, bureaucrats can minimize interactions between clients and the community. The mentally ill remain hidden, under the eye of the Father and away from public attention" (132). Brown and Smith, feminist advocates, also criticize the reproduction of the family in group home settings: "New services have tended to imitate the nuclear family in grouping people together in small houses, [and] women in these groups are likely to find themselves in a housekeeping role ... servicing men whom they have not chosen and with whom they do not have close personal ties" (1992, 159–60).

Group home tenants may indeed constitute family for one another. However, following Fenby (1991), I suggest that including staff in this relationship dynamic would be inaccurate. Relationships between paid staff and tenants are contingent on salary. It has been painful for psychiatric survivors to realize that emotional bonds with staff are time and place specific (Shaunessy 2001). Certainly, "group homes are a risky environment due to frequent changes of staff personnel, high workload of staff, discontinuity in staff presence and limited opportunities for individual support" (Schuengel et al. 2010, 39). Indeed, employee loyalty is to the employer rather than to tenants. It can be dangerous for tenants to rely on paid staff for friendship or emotional support, as there may not be ongoing contact once employees resign.

Critical scholars argue that group homes are mini-institutions (Sinson 1993). Psychiatric survivors and developmentally disabled persons describe a lack of control over their own finances (Sinson

1993), lack of control over choice of roommates (Forester-Jones et al. 2002), strict and inflexible housing rules (Bendell et al. 2010), and staff interference with expression of sexual orientation (Abbott and Howarth 2005). From residents' perspectives, group homes can reproduce aspects of asylum life (Drinkwater 2005).

There must also be a critique of the family as it functions in patriarchal society. The male figurehead who dominates the nuclear family can, as Fenby (1991) suggests, be reproduced by the group home operator as he uses or abuses his power. While the notion of family is used by both group home tenants and the operator to assert their similarity to local inhabitants, the ideal of family itself is problematic. The designation of group home tenants as "family" has implications far beyond the emotional connections that tenants and/or staff may share with one another. First, if municipal government had conceived of tenants as "family," there would have been no public hearing. Indeed, the structure under dispute, which housed sixteen tenants, had previously housed an extended family, also comprised of sixteen people. The structure became the focus of opposition only when the operator applied to open a group home.

The spatial organization of the group home did not reflect what might be considered a typical "family" home in Placeville. While the exterior of the house was home-like by comparison to psychiatric hospitals, interior arrangements revealed aspects of institutional life. Although the operator argued at the O M B that the group home was indeed a home and should not, therefore, be subject to flood plain restrictions pertaining to institutional use, nevertheless the group home manifested several institutional features. For example, an online description of the group home indicated that tenants had to request permission to place computers in their rooms. Adult members of a typical family unit would not have needed such permission. Obtaining operator "approval" infantilized tenants and removed their autonomy.

Similarly, the eating area, as presented in an online image, was inconsistent with the operator's views articulated during the O M B hearing. In a "family" home, the dining room would have had one large table around which everyone sat. In the group home, there were five small tables and, usually, three chairs. Such seating arrangements resembled a restaurant, or perhaps a nursing home environment. The owner also altered the use of transitional and/or recreational spaces. By using the main foyer as an expanded dining area, the operator effectively decreased the common space within the home. Because of decreased space inside, tenants were forced outside if they wished to socialize with one another.

While tenants themselves referred to each other as "family," spatial arrangements within the group home attested to the power exercised by the landlord. Furniture arrangement and use of space demonstrated limited support for tenants' relationships. If development and maintenance of familial links had been a priority, tenants would have been seated around one table and informal social spaces would have been created. The evidence provided at the public meeting and later at the O M B supported the assertion that tenants were "family" to one another. But these relationships appear to be sustained in spite of, rather than because of, the operator's influence.

CONCLUSION

Land use law, which regulates group home location, reflects inherent tensions. On one hand, the group home in this case study was a "residential" use. Nonetheless, it was subject to specific restrictions other "family" dwellings did not face. Since physical structure was not at issue, one can only conclude that psychiatric survivor inhabitants attracted greater scrutiny from the municipality. Tenants' assertion of a family relationship established their dwelling place as a home, a conclusion ultimately supported by the O M B . Despite this concerted effort to assert the centrality of their relationships to one another, the landlord ultimately controlled interior physical space and exerted strong influence on exterior space as well.

Psychiatric survivor resistance to land use law in this case study manifested in two ways. First, survivors identified as a "family," despite its non-traditional nature. Tenants also resisted efforts at visual buffering and the "medical gaze" by their lack of compliance with landscaped terrain outside their home.

Foucault (1984) insisted upon an analysis focused on the centrality of power. He also insisted that such an analysis did not preclude the struggle for social justice. As Foucault famously noted, "liberty is a practice" (1984, 245). It is precisely this analysis of freedom, as a vital force, in action, that encouraged psychiatric survivors to challenge the idea of normalcy itself. It is precisely this analysis of freedom that offered psychiatric survivor tenants the opportunity to reconceptualize themselves, not as loosely connected individuals, but rather, as members of a community.

NOTES

1 Thanks to Jill Grant whose feedback on earlier versions of this chapter helped clarify my arguments and strengthen my writing and to Howard Epstein, whose comprehensive knowledge of land use law guided my analysis of legislation. Thanks also to SSHRC and the Trudeau Foundation who funded the research on which this chapter is based. Finally, I express my deepest appreciation to members of the psychiatric survivor community without whose support I would not have been able to write this chapter.

2 I use this term to indicate that "psychiatric survivors" often survive experiences of oppression, such as sexism, racism, etc., and medicalization of their psychological distress. While the term "psychiatric survivor" can be criticized for defining persons solely in the context of their relations to the psychiatric system, the term has also been used to signal that one has survived one's own psychological distress.

3 This chapter uses a psychiatric survivor analysis to understand the experiences of group home tenants. Psychiatric survivor struggles are also linked more broadly to the struggles of disabled persons. Psychiatric survivors may live with an impairment such as depression or disassociation. Because of the impairment, survivors may also experience disability. For example, a manager may discover that their employee once experienced depression. Subsequently, the employee may be fired because their boss believed they would be unreliable, even if there was no immediate evidence to support their assumption. In the above circumstance, the psychiatric survivor lost their position not because of the impairment, but because of disability i.e. an experience of marginalization due to sanism or systemic discrimination.

4 D. Davidson and M. Lapp, "The Evolution of Federal Voting Rights for Canadians with Disabilities," (2004), http://www.elections.ca/res/eim/article_search/article.asp?id=17&lang=e&. Last accessed 5 November 2012.

5 "At the Asylum," *Globe and Mail*, 5 April 1890.

6 Author unknown, "Seeking House Parents," *Toronto Star*, 16 January 1961.

7 The City of Cornwall amended its group home definition in 2002 to read as follows: "Group Homes" shall be defined as a single housekeeping unit in a single family or semi-detached dwelling in which no more than three (3) (excluding supervisory staff or receiving family) live as a family under the responsible supervision consistent with the particular needs of its residents.

8 In addition to the conflict regarding the application of municipal bylaws, the case revealed a conflict between Placeville's understanding of "group

home" and that of provincial statute. A group home, as defined in the *Municipal Act*, had a maximum of ten tenants. The operator in the O M B case had sixteen tenants. In legal terms, the operator was not operating a group home and could not be found guilty of that offence.

9 No case citation is noted in order to maintain confidentiality of research participants.

10 Members of the queer community use the term "chosen family" to describe those to whom they have no biological relationship but with whom they are deeply bonded. The song "We are Family" by Sister Sledge is particularly popular at gay and lesbian events (Weeks, Heaphy, and Donovan 2001). The song is also mentioned on the website for Family Home Ontario, an organization that links developmentally disabled adults to caregiving families (see http://www.familyhomeontario.org/).

11 Canadian Broadcasting Corporation (C B C), "Manitoba Launches Review of Group Home after Allegations of Abuse," *News Online*, 27 June 2008, http://www.cbc.ca/canada/manitoba/story/2008/06/27/lost-inquiry.html. Last accessed 5 November 2012.

12 "Physicians' Duty to Report Patients," Ontario Ministry of Transportation, 2012, http://www.mto.gov.on.ca/english/dandv/driver/medical-review/physicians.shtml. Last accessed 3 November 2012.

13 E. Reilly, "Council Votes against Group Home Move to Corktown," *Hamilton Spectator*, 26 April 2012, http://www.thespec.com/news/local/article/712656--council-votes-against-group-home-move-to-corktown. Last accessed 4 November 2012.

14 R. Aulakh, "Napanee Group Home Owners File Human Rights Complaint," *Toronto Star*, 7 August 2012, http://www.thestar.com/news/canada/article/1238592--napanee-group-home-owners-file-human-rights-complaint. Last accessed 4 November 2012.

8

Disability, Divisions, Definitions, and Disablism: When Resisting Psychiatry Is Oppressive

A.J. WITHERS

Psychiatric consumer, survivor, ex-patient, and mad (pride) movements have made incredibly important gains for psychiatrized people and for society as a whole. I am personally inspired and influenced by the rich history of psychiatric consumer, survivor, ex-patient, and mad (also known as c/s/x/m) organizing. However, like all movements, there are areas that merit critical re-examination. Geoffrey Reaume (2012), historian and psychiatric survivor, asserts that "being inspired by those who went before can be as good a reason as any to engage in this research, so long as we are also critical about those we may admire, whilst also recording how they made mistakes and could be as offensive as anyone else" (63). I am writing this chapter with critical admiration. This chapter examines sites in which disablism is present in c/s/x/m organizing and calls on organizers to work to undo disablism rather than reinforce it.

I am raising these issues as a physically disabled person[1] in helping to make a useful critical intervention into some problematic tendencies that I have noticed in these movements. I am also psychiatrized as a trans person, because my gender identity is constructed as a mental disorder.[2] I'm writing out of respect and in the hopes that disablism can be eliminated in these movements in order to make them stronger, more inclusive, and more just.

By no means do I intend to suggest that psychiatric survivors, ex-patients, mad people, and/or consumers are not also oppressed by other disabled people organizing for social change. Examples of physically disabled people excluding, erasing, discriminating against, stigmatizing, marginalizing, dominating, or being otherwise oppressive towards psychiatrized people are commonplace. A number of physically disabled people resisted the inclusion of psychiatrized people in the Canadian Charter of Rights and Freedoms (Vanhala 2011). Further, the social model, one of the primary alternatives to the medical model within the disability movement, was not initially developed with psychiatrized people in mind (Oliver 1996). Only after this theoretical model had been elaborated was room made for the inclusion of psychiatrized people (Thomas 2004). I'm not trying to minimize or erase the marginalization of psychiatrized people and psychiatric-survivor perspectives from the disability movement in focusing this chapter on disablism in c/s/x/m movements. Nor am I trying to erase the many times these movements have been hetero-sexist/homophobic, racist, sexist, classist, cissexist, ageist, or otherwise oppressive. Even radical movements led by thoughtful, rigorous, directly affected people have a tendency to reproduce other forms of social/political oppression while they fight to dismantle a particular kind of oppression or gain particular rights.

WHAT IS DISABILITY?

I want to be very clear in what I mean when I say disability. I am invested in the radical model of disability (Withers 2012). Within this framework, disability is about power and oppression; disabled people are labeled as disabled because we are considered un(der) productive within the capitalist economy. Disability is socially specific and has been viewed very differently in different times, places, and cultures. This is how the same person can be labeled as disabled and condemned, stigmatized, and vilified for having visions in one culture but celebrated in another. This is also how a Deaf person can be labeled as disabled in one time and place but in another be viewed as a normal contributor to society (for example, Martha's Vineyard in the early twentieth century [Groce 2003]). Similarly, in a world without stairs, a wheelchair user may not be considered disabled.

There are four key components to the radical disability model. The first is that disability is a social construction not a biological fact. This is not to say that biology isn't at play (we are all biological creatures) but, rather, that we actively attach meaning onto people's minds and bodies. There is no fundamentally biological basis of disability. In the 1970s, physically disabled activists created the social model of disability, separating disability (social barriers) from impairment (physical limitations) (Oliver 1996). The radical model rejects this dichotomy for a number of reasons; particularly, because impairment itself is socially constructed. This isn't to say that disabled people don't have difficulties with our minds and bodies. All humans sometimes have difficulties with our minds and bodies; however, such difficulties are neither a prerequisite nor necessarily sufficient for being categorized as disabled. The radical model is opposed to the medical model of disability. The medical industrial complex, including psychiatry, is fundamentally flawed and perpetuates the oppression of subordinated groups. Condemning this, however, is not condemning the people who access its services nor is it condemning the idea of care.

The second key component to the radical disability model is the idea that disability is about power; as Devlin and Pothier observe, disability "is a question of politics and power(lessness), power over, and power to" (2006, 44). The way that people are categorized as disabled or non-disabled occurs because of the desire to maintain domination over people and control resources. In a capitalist economy these are generally people deemed to be un(der)productive.

Third, disability must be approached from a perspective that recognizes interlocking oppressions. Some members of all subordinated groups are disabled. Eliminating disablism means both working for the elimination of all oppression, and acknowledging that disabled communities are diverse.

Finally, radical access is a key component of radical disability politics. Access becomes much more than physical accessibility and includes, but is not limited to, social, economic, cultural, and intellectual accessibility. The definition of "access" goes beyond the provision of ramps and lifts, towards creating non-oppressive spaces that are inclusive to many different communities (Withers 2012).

DISABLISM IN THE MOVEMENT: LANGUAGE

There are two key ways that I have observed disablism occurring in c/s/x/m movements: the use of disablist language and the reluctance to be called disabled/included in the disability community. When I talk about the way that disability is portrayed by these movements, I do not mean to raise trivial points, or to give credence to the liberal notion of political correctness. Barnes, Mercer, and Shakespeare affirm that "the language and concepts we use influence and reflect our understanding of the social world" (1999, 11). When disability is portrayed negatively, this indicates that disabled people are being undervalued and stigmatized.

Members of the c/s/x/m movement warn of psychiatric drugs and their "brain-disabling" effects (Breggin 1997, 2008), call them "crippling,"[3] and argue they "disable and disempower through their unique disabling effects."[4] Similarly, electroshock is also said to have "brain-disabling" (Breggin 1979) and "disorienting and disabling" (Breeding and Scogin 2012, 60) effects. Activists also called for E C T to be banned because it "frequently causes learning disabilities and other intellectual ("cognitive") impairments" (Psycho U T Conference 2010).[5] Psychiatrists as a whole are said to: "frequently cause harm, permanent disabilities, death – death of the body-mind-spirit."[6] This particular line of discourse is actually doing something quite regressive; it uses a stigmatized identity of one group as shorthand for representing the victimization/disempowerment/oppression of disabled people. This practice ultimately reinforces all disabled people's oppression, which works to reinforce oppression generally.

It is possible that some of these authors are trying to evoke images of disabled people to repel people from psychiatry and/or specific psychiatric interventions. It is also possible that some of these authors would argue that these words, words like "disabling," "crippling," and "impairments" have definitions that do not necessarily imply oppressed identities. However, I think Chris Chapman is correct when he asserts that while words "have acceptable usages about things other than people, in terms of what dictionaries say ... it is impossible to use these words without evoking people." He continues: "whatever dictionaries say – it would be impossible for me to say 'gay' and have it only signify 'happy'" (2010a, n.p.). When arguments are made against psychiatric interventions using this type of language, they are made at disabled people's expense.

Disability, including disabled people, is used as shorthand to represent things that are bad, negative, and undesirable. I do not dispute the fact that there can be awful consequences from psychiatry and psychiatric treatments. I do, however, resent the use of my identity as in need of being prevented and the result of harm. It is important for everyone engaged in these movements (and everyone, generally) to be more intentional with their language. The point of protest is

actually suffering, pain, harm, infringements on autonomy, domination, abuse of power, violence, forced "treatment," and/or
oppression – not disability, or disabled people. Sometimes, this
means using more words and saying the things that are actually
meant rather than using the perceived tragedy of disabled people's
lives as shortcuts.

"WE'RE NOT DISABLED"

The other site where disablism occurs in these movements is through
the conscious distancing of psychiatrized people from disabled communities. I have identified some key themes with respect to why
many psychiatrized people do not identify as disabled: the belief
that disability is "real" and psychiatric diagnoses are not; the belief
in the permanence of disability; the concern about being further
stigmatized; the distancing from and erasure of people labeled as
intellectually disabled; and the belief that psychiatry alone is a form
of social control, to the exclusion of other areas of medicine. While
all of these themes are interrelated and, as I will argue, rooted in
disablism, I will address each one of them individually.

"There's Nothing Wrong with Us"

A common assertion made by the anti-psychiatry movement is that
disability is real and psychiatric diagnoses are not, therefore psychiatrized people are not disabled. For instance, Barbara Everett
argues that adopting, or accepting, the label of disability is inappropriate because psychiatric labels are socially constructed. Everett
asserts, "no one can dispute a developmental handicap or the reality
of the loss of limbs or eyesight. Yet, almost every aspect of mental
illness is contested ground. Some of us even argue that it doesn't
exist" (2000, 199–200). Similarly, Liz Sayce has argued that some
psychiatrized people do not identify as disabled because: "Disabled
people (some user/survivors believe) have a tangible impairment,
for example, being unable to walk or see. A diagnosis of mental illness is much more in the eye of the beholder; it is not clear that there
is something 'wrong'" (2000, 133).

Many psychiatric-survivors, consumers, ex-patients, and/or people who identify as mad are "unwilling to see themselves as disabled.
They associate disability with the medicalization of their distress

and experience. They reject the biological and genetic explanations of their distress imposed by medical experts. They may not see themselves as emotionally or mentally distressed either, but instead celebrate their difference and their particular perceptions" (Beresford, Gifford, and Harrison 1996, 209). Similarly, Recovery Network: Toronto (2012) asserts: "If we hear voices it does not mean that we are ill or disabled – it simply means that we hear voices."[7] Likewise, EleMental, a UK based self-help recovery organization with a presence in Canada and the United States, argues: "Mental distress is not a disability so why try to turn it into one?" These organizations imply that hearing voices and mental distress can be a normal part of the human condition but disability and illness are negative and abnormal.

There are two problematic things that are happening within these lines of argument. First, the maintenance of the myth that disability is fixed and biological is an integral component of maintaining disablism against both intellectually and physically disabled people. Second, these kinds of "we're not disabled because there's nothing wrong with us" statements imply there is something wrong with disabled people. In challenging the pathologization of certain people and certain kinds of pathologies while upholding the systems that allow for and legitimize pathologization, there is a clear effort to distance psychiatrized people from others classified as disabled, leaving disablism intact.

Recovery vs. the Permanence of Disability

Another reason that psychiatrized people resist inclusion within the disability label is the view that disability is permanent. Sayce reports that there is a belief that "Mental distress is not a disability because it is not something that you are born with and it is not permanent; people recover, they are 'survivors'" (2000, 134). EleMental asks: "Why jump on the Disability Rights bandwagon? People can and do recover from mental health problems" (n.d.). This position seems to put forward the idea that disability is inherent to certain individuals. However, most disabilities are acquired rather than inborn.

Even when psychiatrized people do adopt the label of disability, they can still reinforce the notion that disability is inherent to certain people. For instance Gisela Sartori, founder of the Second Opinion

Society, says of her organization, "we came to the point of saying
'Yes. We're disabled; we don't have an inherent disability, but the
system has made some of us disabled'" (in Shimrat 1997, 131)
because of the effects of psychiatric drugs. Even here, where disability is accepted in some circumstances, people reject that psychiatrized people are necessarily disabled while, at the same time,
implying that other disabled people are inherently disabled.

Stigma

Fear of being further stigmatized and marginalized is another reason
that psychiatrized people, mad people, and psychiatric survivors
resist categorization as disabled. Sayce explains this perspective:
"taking on the term 'disability' means taking on another stigma.
Having one stigma is bad enough" (2000, 135). This has been the
position of many in c/s/x/m movements since at least the early 1970s
(Chamberlin 1990). However, this is not how stigma works. People
do not get to choose if they are oppressed – they simply are. Vic
Finkelstein, while writing about a similar pattern of distancing
from the disabled community by the Deaf community, points out:
"Regardless of personal wishes ... being labelled disabled in the
contemporary world is a fact of life for all disabled people" (2000,
268). Like it or not, the disabled identity is not one that is within
the control of most disabled people, and the experience of disablism
certainly is not. This is partly because disability (including impairment) is a social construction, and there are no fixed borders to
determine who is and who is not disabled. You are disabled if you
are constructed as disabled, and stigma and subordination comes
along with that. In addition to the fact that the label "disabled" is
outside the realm of control of psychiatrized people, there is another
serious problem with the attempt to resist additional stigmatization
by not identifying as disabled: simply working to not be considered
disabled in order to avoid stigma without doing anything to a challenge the stigmatization of disabled people is, at best, a demonstra-
tion of a lack of solidarity, and at worst, complicity in oppression.

Erasure of People Labeled as Intellectually Disabled

It is particularly interesting that some c/s/x/m activists endeavor to
unravel the DSM (American Psychiatric Association [APA] 1980,

2000) by working to uphold certain parts of it. I am speaking specifically about the disablism directed at people labeled intellectually disabled. Intellectual disabilities are pathologized through the DSM in the same way that other psychiatric illnesses are named and categorized. However, I could find no discussion of intellectual disability as psychiatrization within c/s/x/m literature. As discussed previously, intellectual disability is named as a consequence of psychiatric treatment – one that should be avoided. In an interview, psychiatric survivor Joe Baletta recounted how he resented his treatment in a psychiatric institution in part because it was assumed people there were "brain dead, retarded, and had no potential."[8] Intellectual disability is also said to be an indisputable reality (Sayce 2000) rather than a social construct – a point disputed by myself and others (Goodley and Rapley 2001, McDonagh 2008, Rapley 2004, Withers 2012).

I suspect that the erasure of this group of people from the movement and community is a direct result of disablism. This disablism is likely functioning both in the belief that people labeled as intellectually disabled are intellectually inferior and in the belief that intellectual disability (diagnoses of mental retardation, learning disorders, etc.) is a wholly biological fact rather than a social construction. Intellectual disability is conspicuously absent in discussions of how the DSM operates to maintain social control within c/s/x/m movement literature.

Medicine as Social Control

Many anti-psychiatry and c/s/x/m organizers argue that psychiatry is used as a tool for social control[9] (see also Breggin 1991, Burstow 2006b, Szasz 1977a). Psychiatric survivor activist Don Weitz asserts that the DSM is a "catalog of negative moral judgments."[10] Subordinated groups, including women (Burstow 2006b, Chesler 2005, Ehrenreich and English 1973), racialized people (Baynton 2001, Greger 1999), Aboriginal people (Dick 1995), poor people (Yolles 1965), queer/lesbian/bi/gay people (Bronski 1984, Foucault 1978, Silverstein 2008), and trans people[11] (see also American Psychological Association 1980, 2000) have been the targets of psychiatric professionals. The pathologization of oppressed groups helps legitimize their oppression, on the grounds that because they are inferior they are in need of special limitations or protections (Ehrenreich and English 1976, Withers 2012).

I have no objection to the argument that psychiatry has been and continues to be used as a tool for social control; I think that is an accurate and important argument. My objection is that people combating psychiatry often imply that psychiatry is socially construed and used for social control while the rest of the medical establishment is helpful, legitimate, not used for social control, and/or based in unbiased science. This is far from the case. While psychiatry has targeted oppressed groups, so, too, has the rest of the medical establishment. Women (Conrad 2007, Ehrenreich and English 1973, Riessman 1998), Aboriginal people (Hoffman 2005), racialized people (British Medical Journal 1901, Haller 1995), poor people (Lidbetter 1921), queer/bi/lesbian/gay people (Ordover 2003, Rahman 2005), and trans (Geddes 2008)[12] people have all been identified as inferior, as disabled, by medical disciplines beyond psychiatry as well.

THE MAINSTREAM GAY RIGHTS MOVEMENT AND RESISTANCE TO PATHOLOGIZATION

A part of winning rights for all of the groups that I listed above has involved distancing themselves from their previous (or current) classification as disabled. One example of this is the mainstream gay rights[13] movement, which worked very hard to distinguish itself from both psychiatrization and disability. This movement serves an example of a campaign against the psychiatrization of (certain) people, and there are a number of parallels between this early anti-pathologization movement and components of contemporary c/s/x/m organizing.

In the 1960s, organized gays and lesbians took an active role in fighting for change. One of the key aims of the struggle was to establish homosexuality as a "minority group" rather than a (psychiatric) disability. Frank Kameny, one of the most well-known American gay rights activists and self-proclaimed founder of the gay rights movement in Washington, DC (Kameny 2009), argued that the categorization of disability needed to become one of the key battlegrounds in the rights movement. Homosexuality had been labeled as a psychiatric illness, or disability, and Kameny, along with the mainstream gay rights movement, organized against the disability or sick label. In a 1964 speech Kameny said: "We cannot ask for our rights from a position of inferiority or from a position, shall I say, as less than whole human beings. I feel that the entire homophile movement, in terms of any accomplishments beyond merely ministering to the needy, is going to stand or fall upon the question of whether or not homosexuality is a sickness, and upon our taking a firm stand on it" (Kameny 1965, 12). This position was echoed by other members of the gay and lesbian community (Esterberg 1990, Silverstein 2008). The mainstream gay rights movement built itself through its separation out from under the disability umbrella.[14]

The APA was (and remains) the gatekeeper of all psychiatric diagnoses and had the power to un-psychiatrize homosexuality. A flier distributed by members of the mainstream gay rights movement reads: "It matters not whether the word used be sickness, disorder, affliction, disturbance, dysfunction, neurosis, immaturity, fixation, character personality disorder, or any other – or whether homosexuality be considered as merely symptomatic of these – the effects are the same: (1) To support and buttress the prejudices of society and to assist the bigots in the perpetration and perpetuation of their bigotry; and, at least equally important (2) To destroy the homosexual's self-confidence and self-esteem, impair his or her self image, degrade his or her basic human dignity."[15] The association of pathologization of identity with the degradation of human dignity is both fair and accurate. However, the authors and protesters consciously associated sickness or disability with the absence of human dignity. This criticism was not of pathologization or the oppressive nature of the classification of disability in general, simply that those in power had erred in classifying them as disabled. This strategy actually worked to maintain disablist oppression and the status quo while negotiating privileged homosexuals' co-optation.

It should be noted that there were some mainstream gay rights activists who did criticize psychiatric pathologization. Charles Silverstein (2008), a gay psychiatrist, presented a paper to the Nomenclature Committee. In it, he argued: "To continue to classify homosexuality as a disorder … is as valid today as was the diagnosis of masturbation in the 1942 edition. What we hope to convey to you is that we have paid the price for your past mistake. Don't make it again" (282). While he criticized psychiatry's moral judgments placed on certain sexual deviancies, he did not apply that criticism to many of the people outside of sexuality and did not question the legitimacy of the American Psychiatric Association or anyone else to pathologize deviant minds and bodies.[16]

In 1973, the mainstream gay rights movement was successful in getting homosexuality delisted as a psychiatric disability. Silverstein called it "the most important achievement of the Gay Liberation Movement" (2008, 227). Homosexuals would no longer be forcibly confined, electro-shocked, drugged, lobotomized, and subjected to other horrors simply for being homosexual. The APA, however, classified sexual orientation disturbance (homosexuality) as a mental disorder when homosexuality itself was removed. Those people who were "disturbed by, in conflict with, or wish[ed] to change their sexual orientation" (1973, 1) were still considered to have mental disorders. Undoubtedly, the depathologization of homosexuality is an incredibly important event in this history, and one that I have personally benefited from; nevertheless, it is important to examine this event critically. It was a victory for many homosexuals at the time but a lot of homosexuals were left behind.

Establishing "ourselves" outside of the rubric of disabled meant that not only did the mainstream gay rights movement sell out its disabled members (not to mention its racialized, poor, trans, intersexed, two-spirited, and, oftentimes, women members),[17] but also that it sold out its future. Fighting to remove itself from the categorization of disabled, rather than working with others classified as disabled to challenge the systems that permit the characterization of undesirable people as disabled, the mainstream gay rights movement has ensured the queer community is at perpetual risk of being repathologized as those in power see fit (the perpetual threat of the discovery of the "gay gene" and subsequent development of prenatal screening of gay fetuses is but one example).

To be gay or lesbian is no longer to be pathological, as white, middle- and upper-class homosexuals and bisexuals, especially gay men, are considered to be productive and useful in contemporary society. The mainstream movement has rallied around assimilationist issues like gay marriage, gays in the military, and adoption that work to uphold capitalist values and social norms. This is done instead of, and at times at the expense of, organizing in defense of "deviant" queer lifestyles like polyamoury, sex work, transsexuality, and genderqueerness that challenge those values and norms. Indeed the actions of the mainstream gay rights movement have, at times, actively marginalized such lifestyles, and the people who choose them.

The struggle to have homosexuality unclassified as a psychiatric disorder was beneficial to homosexuals who were not otherwise psychiatrized or considered disabled. Nevertheless, it's incredibly problematic to purchase privilege at the expense of more marginalized members of the community.

LEARNING FROM HISTORY

I tell this story of the mainstream gay rights movement's co-optation and precariousness because I think there is an important lesson to be learned here about the way the disability movement is approached by those who remain categorized as disabled within broader society. I would argue that c/s/x/m movements are engaging in types of actions that the mainstream gay rights movement engaged in during the 1960s and 1970s, including the use of similar rhetoric. While this strategy could potentially benefit some psychiatrized people, I do not believe that it is in the interest of psychiatrized people as a whole, and it actively works to reinforce the oppression of disabled people.

Let's say for a moment that you aren't buying my argument at all. Let me ask you then, what happens with psychiatrized people who would otherwise be classified as disabled even if psychiatric diagnoses were no longer considered disabilities? Purchasing privilege on the backs of disabled people could actually make many psychiatrized and otherwise disabled people's lives worse. Fellows and Razack argue that "competing parallel narratives ignore the interlocking nature of systems of domination and the complex ways in which they simultaneously secure relations and sites of domination" (1997–8, 339). Separating out psychiatrization from disability and making it a parallel struggle works to erase the ways that interlocking oppression plays out, particularly for psychiatrized and otherwise disabled people.

CONCLUDING THOUGHTS AND MOVING FORWARD

While I have argued for psychiatrized people to identify as disabled and remain under the disability umbrella, I am, nevertheless, conscious of the concerns of psychiatrized people about maintaining their own histories and identities. There are concerns that this could "dilute or co-opt the survivor movement voice."[18] Frank Bangay argues: "While it is important to link up and campaign about issues that affect us all, such as benefit cuts, we need to hang onto our own history and acknowledge our struggle for rights. Otherwise, our views are diluted" (2000, 102). I think that this argument, unlike many of the others, is made in a way that is respectful of disabled people as a whole. I respect this concern. However, I disagree that accepting being labeled as disabled would necessarily mean this loss of history and identity. I believe that a careful, thoughtful, and respectful merger under the rubric of disability can take place without there being a loss to psychiatrized people, including those who identify as mad, psychiatric survivors, ex-patients, and/or consumers.

Unlike the social model, the radical model was developed with psychiatric, intellectual, and physical disability in mind. While the primary developers of this radical model that I am promoting are physically disabled (myself and Loree Erickson), our work was done in close consultation with psychiatrized people, and draws on many of the important contributions that the psychiatric survivor movement has made.

In spite of divisions, there have been important instances of the c/s/x/m organizations and disability organizations working together (Morrison 2003). The Disability Action Group (it later became DAMN), which I was involved with included a number of community organizers, including psychiatric survivors, psychiatrized people, and physically disabled people. This action group had five key demands, including changing certain social assistance regulations, increasing physical accessibility, and eliminating psychiatric abuse.[19] There are undoubtedly many instances of coalitions that emerge out of these communities to work together to achieve specific goals.

Psychiatrized people and members of c/s/x/m movements have the choice to identify as disabled but they do not have choice regarding if they are identified as disabled, nor if they experience disablism. There are only two ways to eliminate disablist experiences of psychiatrized people: to no longer be considered disabled, upholding (even intensifying) the oppression of those disabled people they leave behind; or, to eradicate disablism and the systems of classification that allow some people to be considered unfit, defective, and disabled. Both projects have been struggles for activists and academics for many decades and would, no doubt, take many years, even generations, longer to succeed. The former would require complicity in maintaining the oppression of others and will only be successful if those with power make it so; the latter, however, works towards the liberation of all disabled people and, indeed, all people and, I believe, will be successful – there is no alternative.

NOTES

1   I am using the term "disabled" people because disability is a political action. Disability is imposed upon us, making us disabled people.

2   I am not claiming an "insider" position here, however. Like most trans people I know, the psychiatrization of my trans identity is a relatively insignificant part of that identity.

3   "What's Needed to Improve Mental Health Recovery Rates?" Mind-freedomvirginia 2012, https://lunatickfringe.wordpress.com/2012/02/18/whats-needed-to-improve-mental-health-recovery-rates/. Last accessed 23 August 2012.

4   M. McCubbin, D. Weitz, P. Spindel, D. Cohen, B. Dallaire, and P. Morin, "Submissions for the President's Consultation Regarding Community Mental Health Services," *Radical Psychology* 2, no. 2 (2001): n.p., http://www.radicalpsychology.org/vol2-2/submission-mccubbin.html. Last accessed 14 October 2012.

5   This was the original wording of a draft resolution for the PsychoUT conference. However, it serves as a positive example of how change can happen. A number of us raised the issue during the conference and worked to educate people about how this language was problematic, and ultimately it was changed.

6   "25 Good Reasons Why Psychiatry Must Be Abolished," D. Weitz, n.d., http://www.antipsychiatry.org/25reason.htm. Last accessed 15 July 2012.

7   Recovery Network: Toronto, "Jennifer Hudson Sang Again after Hearing Dead Brother's Voice in Her Head" 2012, http://recoverynetworktoronto.wordpress.com/2012/01/05/jennifer-hudson/. Last accessed 25 August 2012.

8   MindFreedom Personal Story Project, "Personal Stories: Joe S. Baletta," n.d., http://www.mindfreedom.org/personal-stories/balettajoes. Last accessed 15 August 2012.

9   "25 Good Reasons Why Psychiatry Must Be Abolished."

10 Ibid.

11 N. Mulé and A. Daley, "Queer Lens of Resistance: A Critical Anti-oppressive Response to the DSM-V" (proceedings of the PsychoUT

Conference, Toronto, 7–8 May 2010), http://individual.utoronto.ca/
psychout/papers/mule-etal_paper.pdf. Last accessed 14 October 2012.

12 The pathologization of transsexualism is also a good example of the arbitrary divisions between psychiatry and the rest of medicine. It is argued
that there are physical brain differences that are caused by the presence of
a gene that interprets hormones differently than people without this gene
do, and that this gene is (often) linked to transsexuality. This could be
classified as genetics, as endocrinology, as psychiatry, or as other disciplines within medicine.

13 I use "gay rights," "gay and lesbian," and "homosexual" in the historical
discussion because those were the words used at the time. While I most
frequently use queer now, queer had a very different meaning during the
anti-pathologization campaign.

14 It should also be noted that early mainstream gay rights activists did not
just work to establish themselves as non-disabled, but also as white, as
middle/upper class, and as gender normative. Kameny compared gays to
Black people, implying that there were no gay Black people (Kameny
1965). The movement also required people to wear gender normative
business attire (Alwood 1996, Kissack 1995), making it inaccessible to
poor people who didn't have business clothes and marginalizing many
trans and genderqueer as well as women who wanted to wear pants for
either political or personal (or both) reasons.

15 B. Gittings and F. Kameny, "Gay, Proud, and Healthy," *The Kameny Papers*
(n.d.): n.p., http://www.kamenypapers.org/correspondence/gayproudand
healthy.jpg. Last accessed 3 February 2010.

16 Charles Silverstein continued to practice psychiatry.

17 The gay liberation movement, as opposed to the mainstream gay rights
movement, did have an anti-racist, anti-sexist, anti-war, and anti-
consumerist, if not anti-capitalist, platform (Rimmerman 2008).

18 M. McKeown, "Alliances and Communicative Action: One Possibility
for Reframing Theory and Praxis" (paper presented at the Distress Or
Disability?: Proceedings of a Symposium, Lancaster University, Lancaster,
15–16 November 2011 (2011 [1994]): 71), http://www.lancs.ac.uk/cedr/
publications/Anderson_Sapey_and_Spandler_eds_2012.pdf. Last accessed
14 October 2012.

19 "Demands," Toronto Anti-Poverty, n.d., http://torontoantipoverty.tao.ca/
torontoantipoverty.tao.ca/demands.html. Last accessed 12 September
2012.

9

Convention on the Rights of Persons with Disabilities and Liberation from Psychiatric Oppression

TINA MINKOWITZ

This chapter derives from the experience of the author in working on the drafting of the Convention on the Rights of Persons with Disabilities (C R P D). The drafting was an extraordinary experience of cooperation and shared power that is particularly unusual in the experience of users and survivors of psychiatry. The combination of international human rights and a social model of disability that highlights discrimination allowed us to bring into focus the violations we experience, and allowed the other parties involved in the drafting and negotiations process to accept a radical change to international law, which is now working its way into the recommendations of human rights monitoring mechanisms, and into proposals for law reform.

The concept of being persons with disabilities is controversial for survivors of psychiatry since many of us entirely resist mental illness labels. However, the notion of being regarded as persons with disabilities, and discriminated against on that basis, resonates with many of us. Being "regarded as" having a disability is one of the bases for protection against discrimination under the Americans with Disabilities Act, and a similar concept of "perceived" disability exists in international discourse. Furthermore, the prospect of eliminating discrimination, including the laws that have allowed psychiatric incarceration and forced drugging/electroshock, opens up a greater freedom for us to acknowledge a need for reasonable accommodation or support without having to risk destructive, harmful, and violent responses.

Resistance to psychiatry can take many forms, and has taken the form of challenges to the laws that permit psychiatrists to take away our freedom and violate our minds and bodies. In the past, such challenges had failed in the legal arena, at best securing reforms within a framework of overall permission and impunity for acts of psychiatric violence. The non-discrimination principle, coupled with the aspirational quality of the human rights framework ("aspirational" in the sense of seeking a higher good and reaching beyond current political realities), and a politicization of disability that had taken place in an earlier United Nations (UN) process, resulting in acceptance of persons with disabilities as spokespersons and experts on their own needs and interests, were decisive in allowing something different to happen with the CRPD.

ARE WE PEOPLE WITH DISABILITIES?

Disability is a heterogeneous concept, one that comprises many variables such that there can be members of the class of "people with disabilities" whose experience of "disability" has nothing in common. Disability can refer to negative judgments by society about some aspect of a person's way of being in the world, whether physical, mental, or behavioral, as being outside the range of human diversity tolerated in our usual descriptions of what a human being is like.[1] Disability can also refer to a situation in which subjective experience of impairment or limitation is combined with intolerance, failure to accommodate associated ways of being in the world, and failure to meet needs connected with the impairment/limitation, or with this way of being in the world. Both these formulations are legitimate in terms of the social model of disability.[2]

The concept of disability is continually evolving such that being mad, being autistic, being a Down syndrome person, being a Deaf person using sign language and experiencing life within Deaf culture, being a person with any kind of body configuration and body experience, may one day no longer be classified as disability. The concept itself may one day be obsolete. But it has utility as a way of describing a cluster of situations relating to discrimination, the hegemony of "normality" as a value judgment against the full range of human diversity, needs that are not being met in environments designed without appreciation of such diversity, and either subjective experience of limitation or impairment in one's own mind, body, or behavior, or being regarded by others as having such a limitation or impairment.[3]

The value for users and survivors of psychiatry is twofold: to enable us to name the discrimination that predates and underlies psychiatric oppression, and to allow us to stake a claim of dignity in expressing our needs and expecting them to be met as a matter of ordinary human solidarity. Paradoxically in naming the discrimination and calling attention to the needs there is a risk of a discriminatory, violent, and objectifying response, an essentializing of our identity that diminishes our full humanity. This is the challenge faced by every equality-seeking movement and it is not the end of the story but, rather, is an ongoing call for humanity to grapple with injustice.

CRPD STANDARDS AND IMPLICATIONS FOR USERS AND SURVIVORS OF PSYCHIATRY NON-DISCRIMINATION: FORMAL AND SUBSTANTIVE EQUALITY

Human rights norms create positive obligations for countries to safeguard and implement our rights and freedoms, including by changing domestic laws that conflict with these norms. The Convention on the Rights of Persons with Disabilities takes as its starting point that people with disabilities must be guaranteed the same rights and other freedoms as others. In applying this principle to specific rights and freedoms, the CRPD incorporates both formal and substantive equality. Formal equality means that our rights and freedoms must be recognized as a matter of law as being equal to those of others. Any law that establishes inferior rights protection based on a disability, as written or applied, is contrary to this principle.

Substantive equality means that people's diversity needs to be accommodated so as to ensure the practical conditions necessary for enjoyment of equal rights. This principle is violated when a person is expected to conform to a way of being in the world that is impossible for them, as a condition of obtaining access to the means necessary for life, well being, participation in a community or communities, learning, work, and any other activities by which human beings relate to the world. Instead of denying access based on such disqualifications, it is a collective responsibility of society, including those currently being denied access, to use imagination and innovation to create means by which all people can access such basic goods. The capabilities approach developed by Amartya Sen (2009) has contributed to an appreciation of substantive equality, but neither Sen nor his frequent collaborator Martha Nussbaum (2006) has satisfactorily addressed the interplay between formal and substantive equality from a disability perspective. Nussbaum in particular claims that some types of disability, particularly cognitive disability, imply that the individual is no longer entitled to the status of personhood. She situates persons with disabilities as being under conceptual and actual guardianship in a similar way as animals or the natural environment. Her accounts of persons with disabilities all speak of children with developmental disabilities from the standpoint of their families, which is offensive and reinforces negative stereotypes when these accounts are treated as emblematic of the disability experience. A key tenet of the disability rights movement and of all equality-seeking movements is the central position occupied by those with direct lived experience, who represent and speak for themselves.

The CRPD is legally binding on all countries that have accepted its obligations by ratifying it. In addition, the CRPD standards also influence the interpretation of human rights obligations under other treaties that a country may have ratified, and under customary international law. The CRPD represents the most highly developed and focused thinking on the meaning of non-discrimination in situations affecting people with disabilities, and so it is natural for it to be taken as a point of reference and source of authoritative guidance for other human rights mechanisms. Significantly, the CRPD standards and related arguments by users and survivors of psychiatry encouraged the Special Rapporteur on Torture and Other Cruel, Inhuman, or Degrading Treatment or Punishment (SRT) (2008) to formulate detailed standards for recognizing forced psychiatry as torture and ill-treatment, which will be discussed further below.

LEGAL CAPACITY

CRPD Article 12 on legal capacity is designed with both formal and substantive equality in mind.[4] There is the formal equality obligation to recognize that people with disabilities have an equal legal capacity as others to make decisions in all aspects of life. This recognition must be incorporated into law, so that it is no longer possible to deny the legal validity of a person's decision on the basis of disability.

The dual meaning of capacity as intrinsic ability ("capacity to [rationally] understand and appreciate the nature and consequences of a decision") and extrinsic office ("capacity" to be recognized as a valid decision-maker in the eyes of the law) allows for, or intentionally suggests, a blurring of meaning, so that disability is treated as a disqualification for the exercise of fundamental human rights and freedoms. This is what C R P D explicitly rejects, so that there can no longer be a questioning of a person's capacity to make decisions. Instead there must be supportive and cooperative processes whereby all people can explore and act on their own choices.[5]

In addition, there is the substantive equality obligation to make available the support that individuals may need in exercising their legal capacity. Safeguards must be established as well to ensure that support measures do not interfere with the guarantees of formal equality. That is, such measures must respect the individual's autonomy, will, and preferences; supporters must act responsibly, by abstaining from conflict of interest and undue influence; and states must provide for feedback mechanisms to ensure good quality support that is working to meet people's needs.

The practical import of this for people labeled with psychiatric disabilities is greater than it may appear at first glance. Involuntary measures in psychiatry – both detention and forced interventions – are implicitly or explicitly premised on the notion that a person lacks requisite capacity to make a decision. It is difficult to counter such an allegation as an individual, since it is both vague and arbitrary, and amounts to an assertion of authority to determine the validity of another person's choices. Involuntary measures based on this notion that someone else knows better what is for my own good can evoke feelings of shame if I begin to doubt myself as a result, and set up a situation of conflict that is contrary to the good intention to offer help and solidarity. The C R P D recognition of legal capacity without distinction based on disability prohibits forced interventions of all kinds as well as the removal of rights and responsibilities in areas of life such as parenting, voting, legal proceedings, and financial decisions.[6] It respects the "dignity of risk" and assures equality before and under the law and the right to legal recourse against acts of harm.

It can also encourage people to ask for the support that they might want but that they have hesitated to mention because such a request can easily be met with coercion and abuse. If support did not mean giving up rights or freedoms, or giving up power and authority to another person, more of us might feel comfortable asking for it. We already see this happening with practices like Intentional Peer Support,[7] where our community has something to offer the rest of the world from our hard-won experience in promoting positive relationships not based on the deficit of any person, and encouraging mutual learning and growth.

Legal capacity implies taking responsibility for our actions and our decisions. We cannot claim a right to make our own choices, and then object that no one stopped us from doing an act that we later regret. This does not mean that we should accept isolation or an alienated individuality. On the contrary, it increases the importance of developing good, trusting relationships in which people feel free to express concern for each other while maintaining respect for difference and for the ultimately unknowable nature of each human being to every other.

We are responsible for the choices we make and so we need to do our best to be satisfied with those choices. We also are accountable to others for choices we make that limit their choices or that cause harm. For this reason, criminal defenses based on disability, like the insanity defense, need to be abolished in favor of a holistic approach that takes account of all the circumstances of a crime in order to fairly assign blame, and that also takes account of a person's circumstances and needs so as not to impose a sentence that will be disproportionately demanding or harmful for the person to serve.[8]

From a restorative justice perspective, the blame and punishment approach to responding to harms done by any person to another is always harmful and needs to be dismantled.[9] The US penal system in particular has been justly criticized for massively incarcerating African Americans and serving a purpose of racial repression and control (Alexander 2012); it is likely that other countries' systems similarly serve to perpetuate unjust inequalities and do not meaningfully redress the wrongs done to victims. When we open up the question of what constitutes justice in circumstances where extreme mental/emotional states play a role, without relying on an excuse that diminishes the person's legal and social equality and capacity to take responsibility for harm done to others, it helps to make visible the need for a restorative justice approach and contributes to the collective understanding of what restorative justice includes and requires.

It will be important to ensure that restorative justice, prison abolition, and penal reform movements do not uncritically rely on mental health services to meet the needs of those who commit harmful acts for healing and support of their own. Our movement has to become involved in figuring out what really meets such needs, as survivors working with Substance Abuse and Mental Health Services Administration's (SAMHSA) trauma-informed care initiative have begun to do in prisons as well as in mental health settings.[10] Practices like Intentional Peer Support, Hearing Voices Network,[11] and other peer support and peer advocacy work need to be made available and the same critiques we apply to mental health services in general apply here. Mental health courts that shift the question of guilt to a question of "need for services," particularly those that require a guilty plea and can impose a prison sentence should the person stop complying with prescribed treatment, are completely a wrong approach if we are committed to full legal capacity and equal rights. Such courts violate both the right to equal legal capacity (CRPD Article 12) and the right to be free from disability-based detention (CRPD Article 14).

LIBERTY

CRPD Article 14 prohibits deprivation of liberty based on the existence of a disability.[12] Laws and practices that target people for deprivation of liberty based on an alleged disability, such as psychiatric detention and civil commitment, are in violation of this standard and need to be abolished. There is no possibility of saving such laws and practices by including additional criteria such as "danger to self or others," or "need for care and treatment." So long as the detention is limited to people who are alleged to have a disability, it is discriminatory and cannot be sustained. Laws that allow preventive detention for individuals alleged to be dangerous to self or others, or to impose unwanted care and treatment, and that apply to everyone without reference to disability, would also violate CRPD Article 14 if it were shown that the underlying purpose was to continue disability-based detention, or that as applied it actually targeted people with disabilities.

Similarly, it is not enough to provide due process guarantees such as legal representation and a court hearing with the opportunity to cross-examine witnesses (Minkowitz 2011). While there should be remedies to challenge any detention that is committed in violation of domestic or international law (including psychiatric detention, which is per se unlawful under the CRPD),[13] these remedies must preclude the judge having any authority to declare that psychiatric detention is lawful. In other words, once it is demonstrated that a person does not wish to remain in a psychiatric facility, the judge must order his or her release. There also need to be systemic measures put in place to re-orient policies, shift resources to services and supports that meet the CRPD standards and values, re-train professionals and staff working in mental health services, and inform people of their newly recognized rights in the mental health system, so as to prevent the occurrence of detention that might happen despite its being abolished by law.[14]

The Committee on the Rights of Persons with Disabilities has called for mental health services to be based on free and informed consent of the person concerned (Committee on the Rights of Persons with Disabilities 2011a, para 35), in compliance with Article 14. This reading of the article recognizes as a practical matter the unity of psychiatric detention and forced interventions of all kinds, and merges the right to liberty with free and informed consent (Article 25) and the right to exercise legal capacity (Article 12) with regard to all inpatient and outpatient services. It also underlines that mental health services are services, and are therefore not to be used as measures of control or security. Even within a prison setting, mental health services, and housing within a mental health unit, are subject to the person's free and informed consent.[15]

CRPD Article 19 (a) addresses the right to live in the community with choices equal to those of others, guaranteeing the opportunity to choose where and with whom to live on an equal basis, and prohibiting measures that compel a person with a disability to live in a particular living arrangement. This provision prohibits involuntary institutionalization, and regimented group housing, that fails to respect or accommodate individuals' autonomy, choices, dignity, or privacy. In addition, Article 19 (b) and (c) require that a wide range of supports and services be provided to support life in the community and to prevent isolation; and that services available to the general public be open and welcoming of people with disabilities and responsive to their needs.

FREEDOM FROM TORTURE AND ILL TREATMENT, RIGHT TO RESPECT FOR INTEGRITY

The CRPD lays the basis for finding that forced medical interventions constitute torture and ill treatment, but the 2008 report of the UN Special Rapporteur on Torture (SRT) has articulated more detailed standards, drawing on the CRPD as well as the Convention against Torture. CRPD Article 15 directs governments to protect persons with disabilities from torture and ill treatment on an equal basis with others, and makes explicit reference to freedom from non-consensual medical and scientific experimentation, a norm already established in the International Covenant on Civil and Political Rights (1966). Article 16 sets out obligations to prevent and redress all forms of exploitation, violence, and abuse, and Article 17 states that persons with disabilities have an equal right as others to respect for their physical and mental integrity. Article 25 (d) directs that health care be provided to persons with disabilities on the basis of free and informed consent. The Committee on the Rights of Persons with Disabilities has so far addressed freedom from forced psychiatric interventions under Articles 15 and 17. Under Article 15 the Committee has expressed concern about "consistent reports of continuous forcible medication, including neuroleptics" and urged the establishment of voluntary mental health services (Committee on the Rights of Persons with Disabilities 2012, paras 30–1); under Article 17 the Committee has expressed concern about forced mental health treatment and urged the legal abolition of treatment "without the full and informed consent of the patient" (Committee on the Rights of Persons with Disabilities 2011b, paras 28–9).

The Special Rapporteur on Torture adopted a standard first proposed by the World Network of Users and Survivors of Psychiatry[16] in the course of the CRPD drafting process. In this formulation it reads: "Medical treatments of an intrusive and irreversible nature, when they lack a therapeutic purpose, or aim at correcting or alleviating a disability, may constitute torture and ill-treatment if enforced or administered without the free and informed consent of the person concerned" (SRT 2008, para 47). The significance of this standard is that it recognizes the gravity of forced medical interventions in which a person's body, mind, behavior, or consciousness – part of their humanness and unique personhood – is being rejected, objectified, and subjected to violent and non-consensual change. It is a dual violation of autonomy and integrity, as well as the added harm of discrimination, which should result in such interventions being recognized per se as torture (as rape has finally been recognized) under the definition in the Convention against Torture.[17]

As explained by the SRT, that definition contains four elements – severe pain or suffering, intent, purpose, and state involvement (2008, para 46). Both the purpose and intent elements are satisfied when pain or suffering is inflicted on persons with disabilities for reasons based on discrimination. The catalogue of purposes in the CAT definition explicitly lists "reasons based on discrimination of any kind" (2008, para 48); furthermore, intent "can be effectively implied where a person has been discriminated against on the basis of disability" (2008, para 49). State involvement is present in the failure to exercise due diligence to prevent, investigate, prosecute, and punish acts of torture as well as in the direct participation by public officials; a legal framework that permits acts of torture and ill treatment by medical professionals would certainly incur both types of responsibility. The level of suffering may vary case by case, but the combined violation of autonomy and integrity motivated by discrimination is recognized as bringing forced psychiatric interventions in general, including forced drugging and forced electroshock, within the realm of torture and ill-treatment (SRT 2008, paras 39, 40, 47).[18]

The recognition of forced and non-consensual psychiatric interventions as torture represents in itself a step towards reparation of the harm done by these acts of violence. It means that, just as we are claiming the status of moral subjects responsible for our own lives and actions, we are also moral subjects in that acts of harm committed against us by others must be accounted for and not trivialized or rationalized away as "therapeutic necessity"[19] or being "for one's own good." It may be a symbolic achievement and cannot stop there; recognition of harm does not by itself stop the harm from continuing. But it remains significant as a beacon of hope for social and legal change, all the more so because it responded to the call from our own community by hearing and embracing our expressed needs.

REMEDY, REDRESS, REPARATION, RESTORATIVE JUSTICE: WHAT MUST BE DONE?

CRPD Article 4 on general obligations requires governments to abolish laws and practices that constitute discrimination against persons with disabilities, to enact new laws, and to take a variety of other measures to ensure "the full realization of human rights and fundamental freedoms for all persons with disabilities without discrimination of any kind on the basis of disability." Article 8 mandates awareness-raising campaigns to combat stereotypes and bigotry, and other action-oriented obligations appear throughout particular articles. In carrying out these obligations, governments must closely consult with the representative (democratic) organizations of people with disabilities, including children with disabilities (CRPD 2007, art 4.3), and they must also establish focal points for implementation and one or more independent monitoring bodies at the national level (CRPD 2007, art 33).

The undertaking of CRPD implementation, both by governments and by civil society, can be approached in a spirit of restorative justice, particularly in relation to ending psychiatric oppression.[20] The oppression has been and continues to be institutional and systemic; countless individuals have been involved as victims, oppressors, and bystanders. We need a healing that ends the power of the psychiatric "parallel state"[21] and that puts law and resources in the service of human dignity. This would have to be a decisive step, eliminating the laws permitting psychiatric detention and compulsory treatment and putting in place effective remedies against the continuation of these abuses. As part of the healing process, an "appreciative inquiry"[22] could be undertaken to understand the nature and scope of harms suffered at the hands of psychiatric oppression, and to invite those who have committed acts of harm to offer their apologies, to demonstrate a new unity of solidarity and reject paternalism. We would want to honour the lives, struggles, and voices of those who have been harmed by psychiatry, and make space for a new way of listening to these stories and absorbing their lessons.

Good faith needs to be demonstrated at the outset or developed in the course of the work so that survivors of psychiatric oppression, including people currently resisting and/or being victimized, do not give up their independence or their moral power to accept or reject any course of action proposed by others. It is only when the system of forced psychiatry is ended – when it is deprived of legal permission and the backing of state power – that any legitimate "truth and reconciliation" can take place, and all participants in any commission overseeing the "appreciative inquiry" would be expected to admit to their own participation in abuses and to not currently be involved in any psychiatric oppression, force, or coercion. There are other ways implementation can happen, of course – including large-scale consultation and reforms without an explicit reconciliation process – and in most countries the reality is likely to be piecemeal struggle through legislation, litigation, human rights monitoring, publicity campaigns, alliance-building, and strategy. A restorative/ reconciliation approach is an option that would be conducive to the involvement of ordinary people who have been harmed and continue to be harmed by psychiatric oppression, and, by receiving the stories and supporting people through the telling, could also contribute to building the social capacity to do things differently.

IMPLICATIONS FOR RESISTANCE

The CRPD, created as a labour of love and pragmatism, unites many seeming opposites: human rights and social development, autonomy and solidarity, equality and diversity, freedoms and entitlements. The elements of legal capacity, liberty, and freedom from torture, which defined the human rights advocacy by users and survivors of psychiatry for the CRPD, are united in the call for restoration of our capacity as moral subjects in the eyes of the law and justice. Bringing justice to justice, a fundamental aspect of equality and non-discrimination, has begun to be accomplished; next, the restoration of justice needs to move from the realm of international law to the national and local plane, and to be experienced in our ordinary lives.

The potential of the CRPD can only be fulfilled when users and survivors of psychiatry and our allies actively organize and advocate for it to be put into practice. The first step is to make people aware that this treaty exists. It is also essential to ensure that it is being interpreted correctly by relevant decision-makers such as government agencies, legislatures, courts, and human rights monitoring mechanisms. In addition, we need to develop proposals for law reform, including the repeal of mental health laws authorizing involuntary commitment, forced interventions, and substituted decision-making.

We can also utilize human rights monitoring mechanisms to put pressure on national governments to take required action.

For these purposes, I established a user/survivor-run human rights organization, the Center for the Human Rights of Users and Survivors of Psychiatry (CHRUSP 2009). CHRUSP contributes to ongoing international advocacy by the World Network of Users and Survivors of Psychiatry, advises user/survivor organizations and allies in all parts of the world, and conducts more focused activities in the United States, where it is based. CHRUSP initiated a call for a Campaign to Repeal Mental Health Laws[23] in the US and Canada, which operates as an independent collective of concerned activists pursuing the goal of repealing these laws and abolishing forced psychiatry. Members of the Campaign are working on human rights reporting to the UN, a Coming Out Campaign, informal outreach, involvement with US ratification of the CRPD and Canadian consultations on implementation, and developing proposals for law reform. There is also a "Repealing Mental Health Laws" group on Facebook[24] for related discussions.

Colleagues in other countries have taken up the challenge and opportunities created by the CRPD, pursuing law reform, human rights reporting, awareness-raising, and campaigns for CRPD ratification. We have benefited greatly from the work of users and survivors of psychiatry who were elected to serve as members of the Committee on the Rights of Persons with Disabilities, and have helped to ensure that the Convention is interpreted according to its intention and principles, requiring the abolition of forced psychiatry and the development of support that respects individual autonomy. It is essential for us to exchange information, knowledge, and strategy ideas. Similarly to the Occupy movement, this work is founded on principles that need to develop and evolve over time and in different local circumstances to see their full fruition. I have every hope and expectation that our resistance will wear away the tyranny of psychiatry as a parallel state and we will succeed in its abolition.

NOTES

1 For example see "Psychosocial Disability," World Network of Users and Survivors of Psychiatry, 2009, www.chrusp.org/media/AA/AG/chrusp-biz/

downloads/199123/Psychosocial_disability.docx. Last accessed 22 October 2012.

2　For example see United Nations (2007, art 1).

3　The inclusion of those "regarded as" having a disability as persons with disabilities, and/or as protected against disability-based discrimination, can be found in the *Americans with Disabilities Act* (2009, 42, s12102), the *Inter-American Convention on the Elimination of All Forms of Discrimination Against Persons with Disabilities* (1999, art 2.a), AG/RES. 1608 (XXIX-O/99), Art 2(a), and the *International Classification of Functioning, Disability, and Health, Short Version* (2001, 27).

4　Paragraphs 1, 2, and 5 of Article 12 mandate formal equality; paragraph 3 mandates substantive equality, and paragraph 4 attempts to reconcile them. In its origins, paragraph 4 drew on safeguards relevant to both substituted decision-making and support, but the guarantee of formal equality and the obligation to respect the person's will and preferences rule out substituted decision-making, as also recognized by the Committee on the Rights of Persons with Disabilities (2007 para 34).

5　See materials on legal capacity through page links "Resources," "More Resources," and "Good Practices" at www.chrusp.org.

6　See CRPD (2007) Articles 23, 29, 13, and 12.5 respectively. The CRPD articles supporting prohibition of forced psychiatric interventions, Articles 14, 15, 16, 17, 19, and 25 are discussed below.

7　"Peer Support and Peer Run Crisis Alternatives in Mental Health," Shery Mead Consulting, n.d., www.mentalhealthpeers.com. Last accessed 22 October 2012.

8　See materials on prison issues through page links "Resources" and "Good Practices" at www.chrusp.org. See also Office of the High Commissioner for Human Rights (2009, A/HRC/10/48, para 47).

9　Restorative Justice comes in many guises (McCaslin 2005, Pranis 2007, Sullivan and Tifft 2001, Tutu 1999). For a cautionary note from a feminist perspective, see Daly and Stubbs 2005.

10　I consider SAMHSA's materials and approach (http://www.samhsa.gov/nctic/trauma.asp) to be of mixed value but worth knowing.

11　"The International Community for Hearing Voices," *Intervoice*, http://www.intervoiceonline.org. Last accessed 22 October 2012.

12　Article 14:

　　1 States Parties shall ensure that persons with disabilities, on an equal basis with others:

　　(a) Enjoy the right to liberty and security of person;

(b) Are not deprived of their liberty unlawfully or arbitrarily, and that any deprivation of liberty is in conformity with the law, and that the existence of a disability shall in no case justify a deprivation of liberty. 2 States Parties shall ensure that if persons with disabilities are deprived of their liberty through any process, they are, on an equal basis with others, entitled to guarantees in accordance with international human rights law and shall be treated in compliance with the objectives and principles of the present Convention, including by provision of reasonable accommodation.

Of particular relevance are paragraphs 1 (b) and 2, which deals with rights in the context of criminal arrest and prison, and other deprivations of liberty. The whole article is copied here for reference.

13 See Article 13 on access to justice, which arguably gives rise to the right to a remedy; see also International Covenant on Civil and Political Rights (1976), Articles 2.2, and 9.

14 See Article 4 (a), (b), (c), (d), (e), (h), and (i), Article 8, and Article 16.

15 See materials on prison issues through page links "Resources" and "Good Practices" at www.chrusp.org. See also Office of the High Commissioner for Human Rights (2009, A/HRC/10/48, para 47) and United Nations (Committee on the Rights of Persons with Disabilities 2011a, para 35).

16 "Contribution by World Network of Users and Survivors of Psychiatry (WNUSP)," World Network of Users and Survivors of Psychiatry, 2004, http://www.un.org/esa/socdev/enable/rights/wgcontrib-wnusp.htm. Last accessed 22 October 2012.

17 That definition reads:

For the purposes of this Convention, the term "torture" means any act by which severe pain or suffering, whether physical or mental, is intentionally inflicted on a person for such purposes as obtaining from him or a third person information or a confession, punishing him for an act he or a third person has committed or is suspected of having committed, or intimidating or coercing him or a third person, or for any reason based on discrimination of any kind, when such pain or suffering is inflicted by or at the instigation of or with the consent or acquiescence of a public official or other person acting in an official capacity. It does not include pain or suffering arising only from, inherent in, or incidental to lawful sanctions. (Convention Against Torture, 1984: art 1)

18 See also in 2008 SRT details on electroshock, forced psychiatric interventions, and involuntary commitment (paras 61–5), medical context

including experimentation (paras 57–60), and less satisfactory details on "prolonged" restraint and solitary confinement (paras 55–6).

19 The European Court of Human Rights adopted this standard in rejecting the claim that being forcibly drugged with neuroleptics and handcuffed to a "security bed" amounted to torture or ill treatment (Herczegfalvy v. Austria, 1992).

20 Given the widespread and systematic practice of serious violations amounting to torture and ill-treatment, remedy and reparation are due under the Basic Principles and Guidelines on the Right to a Remedy and Reparation for Gross Violations of International Human Rights Law and Serious Violations of International Humanitarian Law, A/RES/60/147 (2006).

21 For a useful analogy see Romany 1994.

22 A term that has been used in the context of Intentional Peer Support.

23 "Repeal Mental Health Laws," 2012, http://repealmentalhealthlaws.org/. Last accessed 22 October 2012.

24 "Repealing Mental Health Laws," *Facebook*, n.d., http://www.facebook.com/groups/356040824414503/?fref=ts. Last accessed 30 September 2012.

10

Deeply Engaged Relationships: Alliances between Mental Health Workers and Psychiatric Survivors in the UK

MICK MCKEOWN, MARK CRESSWELL,
AND HELEN SPANDLER

INTRODUCTION

This chapter explores the possibility of alliances between mental health workers and psychiatric survivor movements – a focus that has received little scholarly attention to date. Particular attention is paid to alliances between survivors and public sector trade unions in the UK. These alliances are replete with what, in a more general context, Wendy Brown (2000) has called *perils* and *possibilities*. The possibilities of such alliances will be framed in terms of the need to defend, as well as transform, health and welfare institutions from threats presented by neoliberalism and bio-psychiatry, as well as the need for a creative renewal of the activism of both the labour and survivor movements. Models of reciprocal community trade unionism and relational organizing will be presented as a potential way of developing "deeply engaged" and reciprocally beneficial relationships (Tattersall 2006) that, we believe, are necessary for the transformation of the mental health system.

We argue that the formation of survivor and worker alliances opens up the sort of communicative spaces wherein an alternative politics of mental health might be realized. Of course, this is not the only way, and we want to be clear that we fully support the importance of the autonomous organizing of psychiatric survivors as well as alliances that reach beyond workers and trade unions to incorporate the lessons of, for example, feminism and recent Occupy movements. Indeed, as will become clear, we are acutely aware that it has been the failings of trade unionism, often attributed to a narrow perspective of "workerism," hierarchy, and bureaucratization, that helped precipitate the growth of single-issue based and identity-focused "new social movements" in the first place (Habermas 1981).

At the same time, we think there are particular perils, and yet enormous possibilities, to be derived from alliances between survivors and mental health workers. These alliances are important for a number of reasons. We believe that there is great potential for personal and wider social change, as well as reciprocal benefit, from both formal and informal alliance-formation. We know that it is often the relationships forged (or neglected) between workers and survivors that are at the heart of people's experiences of the mental health system – whether these experiences are profoundly positive or negative. Indeed, front-line workers are often seen as the bearers of a rightly maligned bio-psychiatry and, as such, often bear the brunt of survivors' critique. However, we think it is important to see workers as potential allies, not least because of the interdependency of workers' and survivors' interests and the fact that, often, both can feel alienated by their experience of the mental health system and, therefore, have a reciprocal interest in its democratic transformation.

Despite this, recent examples of formal alliances involving public sector trade unions and survivor groups are actually quite rare, and, when they do occur, they are as likely to bring out tensions in the relationships as any easy solidarity. In this chapter, therefore, we draw together some examples from England which illustrate some specific perils and possibilities. These include reflections on the establishment of the London Mental Patients Union in the 1970s (Spandler 2006); a social services strike in Sheffield in the early 1990s (Cresswell 2009); and, more recently, a mental health nurses' strike in Manchester in 2007 (McKeown 2009). Whilst these illustrate what might be called "imperfect solidarity,"[1] it is a solidarity we argue is ever more urgent in the context of neoliberal threats to the provision of welfare. Despite, or perhaps because of, the challenges involved, we offer an optimistic analysis that sees possibilities in even the perils and always considers the implicit potentiality and creativity of community campaigning, political, and industrial action.

However, we want to be clear about one point, despite our optimism. To talk about the perils and possibilities of alliance-formation between survivors and workers is not the same as invoking the politics of mental health as a *level* playing field in which the power and knowledge wielded by workers, on the one hand, and survivors, on the other, is, in practice, equal. We fully accept that what characterizes the politics of mental health is a certain "legitimation crisis" (Habermas 1976) in which the power and knowledge of workers has been systematically portrayed as legitimate and objective ("reasonable") and the power and knowledge of survivors has been historically subjugated as "mad." This crisis profoundly structures the politics of mental health and addressing it, therefore, is a precondition for any democratic alliance worthy of the name. In other words, sustained joint action between labour and movements of psychiatrized people depends on a profound challenge to prevailing understandings of "mental illness" or "madness" *and* a shift in the power relations between survivors and professionals. Any alliance that simply reinforces the power of the psychiatric profession is not what we seek. An appreciation of these issues underlines our contribution. It is also one of the reasons why we refer to psychiatric "survivors" throughout this chapter (rather than mental health "service users" or "consumers").

ALLIANCES IN ACTION: THREE UK EXAMPLES

One of the authors here, Mark Cresswell, was a trade union activist for NALGO,[2] during a long, hard-fought strike in Sheffield's social services in 1991 (see Harrison 1992). The dispute was over pay, conditions, and adequate access to training opportunities for Residential Social Workers. A clear asset of this struggle was the degree of solidarity demonstrated between the local survivor groups and the striking workers. This solidarity was no accident, neither was it what Amanda Tattersall (2006, 590) has called an "ad hoc relationship" or a "simple coalition"; rather, it was more of a "deeply engaged relationship." In fact, this relationship had been forged over many years by a highly committed and powerfully unionized team of mental health workers connecting with a historically established, strong organization of survivors. One of the most spectacular features of the dispute – certainly the one that received the most, and most sympathetic, media attention – was that a group of survivors entered and occupied one of the vacant premises, continued to make it available during the dispute, and were supported by striking workers with food parcels and moral support. The survivors and the strikers were, nevertheless, understandably worried that management might use the strike opportunistically as an excuse to cut services and close buildings.

On returning to work after seven months out, the workers found a new and curious power dynamic in their relationships with survivors. One might reasonably have expected a state of enhanced reciprocity. Some of the survivors, however, especially those who had been most active during the strike, began to question, at the most basic level, their actual need for the services provided by the workers – the very services that they had fought so hard, so recently, to defend. After all, survivors argued, we demonstrated as much organization as you without the resources of a trade union behind us; we demonstrated as much ingenuity as you and we're supposed to be "mad"; we demonstrated as much self-determinism as you and we're supposed to lack energy and direction. Could not these very qualities be indicative of mental well-being rather than "madness"? Why should we now be considered as somehow dependent upon you? What, then, is the point of this job of yours, which we've all fought so hard to defend? Why should you get a pay packet every month – *now*, an enhanced pay packet – and we, if we're lucky, get Disability Living Allowance?

This was a challenge that certainly caused some consternation amongst the workers and the union activists. The productive compromise reached was that more autonomous spaces were provided within local authority premises for survivors to run survivor-only groups. Day Centres, for instance, after much negotiation, were made available for survivors to use at weekends without workers present. This meant quite radical innovation for the time such as, for instance, providing survivors with their own sets of keys. Such measures, however, in no way fully responded to the sheer *depth* of the survivors' critique.

A similar, but earlier dispute helped to lay the seeds for a radical Mental Patients Union (MPU) to emerge in the 1970s. This was formed in the context of action in 1972 to defend Paddington Day Hospital in London from closure. The social history of these important events has been explored in some detail (Crossley 1999,

Spandler 2006, Survivors History Group 2012) – but a couple of points are worth revisiting here. The service under threat was a therapeutic community, and the forms of libertarianism and the democratization of social relations it represented were important precipitants for the alliances between workers and survivors that were to evolve in the course of the campaign. Having said that, it is important to recognize that therapeutic communities did not *necessarily* provide an environment that allowed survivor power to develop, and conversely less democratic services did not necessarily prevent it. Whilst the events in London may have helped raise the profile of this emerging new movement, the first signs of a Mental Patient's Union happened in a Scottish asylum in 1970.[3] Perhaps the interesting point here is that, whilst the Scottish Union was developed by survivors autonomously, in solidarity with each other, the London MPU was initiated by an alliance between survivors *and* workers who together had forged links with other progressive political groups and movements[4] (see also Crossley 1999, Spandler 2006). This connection with, for example, the organized left was, however, quite limited (especially once the campaign had died down) and, despite representations by MPU members, the Trades Union Congress refused to recognize it or allow it to affiliate as a "genuine" union (as patients were not workers).

A key issue that arose after the largely successful campaign was that the service became gradually removed from what survivors had originally been fighting for. In a bitter and ironic turn of events a few years later (detailed in different ways by both Baron 1987, and Spandler 2006) some of the survivors were actually involved in complaints *about* the day hospital itself and it eventually closed down. Whilst the merits, and indeed, the democracy of therapeutic communities are often contested by radical survivors, it is perhaps unfortunate that therapeutic communities are now few and far between in current mental health provision in the UK where reciprocal learning and alliances can potentially flourish.

In another more recent dispute, mental health nurses in Manchester took strike action as part of a wider campaign to defend services from cuts and, specifically, to seek the reinstatement of the psychiatric nurse and union activist Karen Reissman, who was sacked for whistle-blowing management's plans for the "reorganization" of (i.e. cuts to) services (McKeown 2009). This dispute illustrates some key issues for trade unions in their appreciation of the politics of mental health. The union's critique of marketization was well argued and the activist's dismissal, which was clearly ideologically driven, needed opposing.

However, the potential for broader alliances between the union and the wider survivor movement was limited by a number of factors. First, the union activists' critique of the "cuts" rather too readily accused the Mental Health Trust of "privatization" when it awarded a mental health service contract to a voluntary sector provider, outside the National Health Service (N H S). This organization, unlike many State-run services, had actually forged good links with local survivors and was subsequently well-liked, as, indeed, was Reissman herself.

Second, despite genuine efforts to form an alliance with local survivors, more broad-based reciprocity with other activists in the region was potentially damaged by failing to challenge some of the ubiquitous discourses about "risk" and mental health. On the whole, the struggle to defend services was covered positively in the local media, as was the alliance with survivors. The media and the campaign, however, also reinforced a number of stereotypes, including articles suggesting the services were primarily needed to protect the public from "dangerous" individuals or portraying survivors as vulnerable and passive and, therefore, in need of expert care. These media representations jarred with the actuality of dynamic survivors demonstrating political agency in support of the workers, participating in rallies, and speaking with conviction from public platforms. One explanation for why the striking nurses did not oppose the media output is that this portrayal of survivors actually served the interests of the strikers (and to a lesser extent the survivors themselves): public fear or uncritical compassion for "vulnerable people" was easily translated into popular support for the strike and a defense of valued workers and services. However, more broadly, these kinds of representations may be seen as collusions that ultimately damage the potential for alliances with more radical members of the survivor movement who seek to more deeply challenge our understandings of madness.

Third, as with many disputes like this, a lack of prior engagement with survivor knowledge and experience limited the depth as well as breadth of potential alliances (Church 1995). The necessity of prior engagement stresses the need to build alliances carefully *before* they can ever be mobilized in the service of reciprocally meaningful action (Wills and Simms 2004). Such circumstances, wherein opportunities to advance more complex but progressive values in action are constrained, have been described in terms of "imperfect solidarity."[5] On the positive side, the alliances that were forged during the dispute have continued to be nurtured and drawn upon in the context of united campaigns against more recent cuts to, and reorganization of, local mental health services. This brings us to the need to understand the broader landscape for alliances in the UK, against an economic backdrop dominated by neoliberalism. This context presents a number of threats to the politicization of both union and survivor organizations, and as such, demonstrates why such alliances are increasingly challenging but remain no less important as a result.

THE NEOLIBERAL CHALLENGE
TO ALLIANCE FORMATION

The last thirty years have ushered in the ascendancy of a neoliberal project that presents a number of challenges, as well as opportunities, for worker and survivor alliances. The first challenge is the sustained attack on welfare provision in the UK and the rise of marketization and privatization. After all, minimizing state welfare provision is at the very heart of neoliberalism. The welfare state in general, and the National Health Service (NHS) in particular has, arguably, never been so vulnerable as it is now to what Colin Leys (2003) has referred to as "market-driven politics" – a sub-set of which Alyson Pollock (2004) has dubbed, sardonically, "NHS plc." The relentless individualization of current policy in health and social care undermines a commitment to the collective provision of welfare. This is a peril that Peter Sedgwick (1982) clearly anticipated in his ground-breaking book *Psychopolitics* and is a core political feature of what Stuart Hall once called "the great moving right show" (Hall 1979).

As we have seen from our examples above, many survivor mobilizations in the UK have actually occurred *in defense of* particular mental health services. This is likely to continue in the years ahead, even though those services are far from ideal. In addition to fears for the future of services, many psychiatric survivors and disabled people face a concomitant assault on their right to welfare benefits. This stark reality represents a possibility for workers and survivors to find common cause in the defense of the NHS and wider welfare provision, and developing links with other social movements, especially the disabled people's movement (Morris 2011). For example, the "Hardest Hit" campaigns, Mad Pride, and UK Uncut have organized joint actions with Disabled People Against Cuts and these kinds of examples are important because they unite the interests of survivors and disabled people and connect with the wider anticapitalist movement (see, for example, *Asylum Magazine* 2012).

Closely connected to the undermining of collective welfare provision has been a sustained attack on the organized labour movement. In the last years we have witnessed steep decline in the numbers of people belonging to trade unions in the UK, particularly in the traditional manufacturing heartlands of unionism. Public sector trade unions, however, such as those operating in health and social care, have remained comparatively resilient. Indeed most of the largest UK trade unions are now to be found in the public sector; the biggest of these, Unison, claims 1.3 million members. In parallel, the public sector now accounts for the majority of industrial action with 59% of all stoppages (Office for National Statistics 2012). Because of these trends, public sector unions are seen as central to the wellbeing of the wider UK labour movement. However, new systems of external commissioning of services mean that, increasingly, many mental health workers are atomized with a resulting tendency for workers to prioritize their individual survival, or the development of their professional careers, over collectivism. While much of the newer mental health workforce is un-unionized, the industrial power of NHS mental health nurses is arguably diluted by divided membership, with large numbers belonging to professional associations rather than unions (Hart 2004).

This same period of turbulence for trade unions has been accompanied by the rise of consumerist policies in health and social care that, ostensibly, urge greater public participation and "service user involvement" (Barnes and Cotterell 2012, McKeown and Jones 2014). Although this opens up important opportunities for survivors to have more of a voice, consumerist rhetoric is often cynically mobilized to undermine workers (and arguably survivor's) collective interests. Indeed, it may be argued that the neoliberal project is precisely what social movements in general, and survivors in particular, have been "co-opted" into. In the UK, first New Labour and now the Conservative-led Coalition have finessed a process of incorporation, which deploys ostensibly progressive rhetoric – such as *user involvement, choice, independence, social inclusion, and recovery* – but this has effectively become an ideological smoke-screen for the neoliberal project. Survivors who do get "involved" have arguably been pulled into the orbit of the powers-that-be – what Michel Foucault (1991b) and others (see Jessop 2007) have called the sphere of governmentality. The threat here is of co-option, of being drawn into the very system that is being challenged so that resistance is neutralized and nullified (Cooke and Kothari 2002, Morris 2011, Pilgrim 2005). Indeed, studies of "user involvement" inside the mental health system have shown that the degree of democratization is limited and that many important topics of impor-tance to survivors do not even make it onto official agendas (Hodge 2005, 2009; Godin et al. 2007). Yet, at the same time, the invitation for survivors to express their demands within services and policy bureaucracies has raised the possibility for more radical voices in the wider movement to begin to infiltrate these settings, squeezing through the cracks of power to raise the standard for more demo-cratic control.

Another challenge to alliances is the pull in the direction of a legal and negative defense of human rights, a situation that Wendy Brown has called the peril of "the transposition of venue from the streets to the courtroom" (2000, 230). So, what begins as collective action for wider societal change can become reduced to legalistic and indi-vidualized tactics alone. Whilst clearly important, legal frameworks have their limitations because their defensive focus on individual "negative rights" tends to obscure the issue of "rights" being located in the wider context of *interdependence* with others. Opposition to enforced treatment, or advocating for "due process," is insufficient if such arguments are not accompanied by a concomitant demand for meaningful alternatives, such as the "minimal medication" approaches, survivor-led crisis houses, and non-medical sanctuaries, that survivors have long demanded (Spandler and Calton 2009). Progressive though it may at times be, the "transposition ... from the streets to the courtroom" must, therefore, be placed within the political context of demands for public assistance and collective provision. This is one of the critiques leveled at the United Nations Convention on the Rights of Persons with Disabilities (UNCRPD) by some survivor activists.[6] Whilst the UNCRPD has rightly been lauded as a ground-breaking legal framework against detention and coercion, it arguably lacks sufficient commitment to "positive rights" (e.g. to support and sanctuary). This is another agenda around which workers and survivors could collectively mobilize.

It is worth noting that the ongoing global financial crisis has been a persuasive *in vivo* test of the inadequacies of the neoliberal project – even as this ideology continues to underpin the economic programmes of governments in the Global North (Quiggin 2010). Crouch (2011) sees the hegemony of neoliberalism as explicable via an analysis of a constellation of political elites, multinational corporations, and mass media conglomerates that are its props. The conspiratorial flavour of this is reflected in analysis of the behind-the-scenes plotting to introduce market forces and privatizations into the NHS, which is mostly hidden from the electorate (Leys and Player 2011). Faced with such evidence, any who would resist may be forgiven for taking the pessimistic view that the neoliberal project is both omnipotent and omnipresent. More optimistically, however, John Clarke (2007) looks for the very places and spaces where neo-liberalism *is not* omnipresent, and finds numerous examples of what he refers to as recalcitrance: as a precursor to political strategies of transformation and resistance. One way to mobilize recalcitrance is to configure alternative forms of worker/survivor alliances. With this in mind, the next section reflects on the value of what has been called reciprocal community trade unionism.

RECIPROCAL COMMUNITY ORGANIZING

The necessity for trade unions to resist neoliberalism has meant that optimizing their organizing capacities has become a key goal (Bach 2010, Gall 2009). One simple strategy for union renewal is to con-centrate on building supportive relationships *within* the union itself. For Paul Jarley, such solutions need to "recreate community in the workplace" by focusing on people rather than issues and building "personal relationships among all members of the work group in ways that create an emotional bond among the workers" (2005, 12–13). A notable model for this is the relational organizing approach patented by the US *Harvard Union of Clerical and Technical Workers*[7] (see also Hoerr 1997). We should be critical, however, of unions that only look inwards to improve their organiz-ing (see Jarley 2005). While this might improve ties between mem-bers, it misses the opportunity to reach beyond the workplace.

Interestingly, after winning famous victories in organizing at the university, the Harvard workers turned to the nearby hospital and formed an effective alliance with service users under the reciprocal slogan: *Pro-Patient, Pro-Union.*

Organizing initiatives that focus only on workplace issues are vulnerable to fluctuations in effectiveness that vary with the rhythms of employer behaviour and may fail to reflect the full range of worker interests, let alone community concerns. It is not too great a leap to extend this philosophy to the desirability of achieving close relational ties and reciprocity with community activists external to the workplace. Therefore, various authors have promoted models of reciprocal community unionism for achieving such alliances between trade unions, community groups, and social movements (see Simms and Holgate 2010, Tattersall 2010, Wills and Simms 2004). For our purposes, this must include engaging with the psychiatric survivor movement, including those who are seen as critical of the workers that trade unions represent. Such reciprocity is predicated upon a commitment to democratic dialogue in which workers engage with survivors and vice versa. In other words, any alliance between workers and survivors needs to be, by definition, *relational* and *reciprocal* although crucially, we would argue, not *symmetrical.* Such asymmetry arises because the politics of mental health is not a level playing field; relationality and reciprocity must always be predicated upon the privileging of survivor knowledge and experience before that of workers. But, to further complicate matters, neither can we assume that "survivor knowledge" is necessarily homogenous or united. This is why genuinely democratic dialogic relations with survivors is such a challenge for workers and why its pursuit ushers in distinctive "perils and possibilities."

In effect, survivors have announced that they will not be passive recipients of welfare; that they will not be dependent citizens; that they demand a voice in the services that are provided for them; and that those services must refuse to stigmatize them. Accompanying such demands will be a multitude of experiences of psychiatric oppression for which the movement seeks both redress and justice. Therefore, one of the *perils* that emerge for trade unionists in the attempt to forge reciprocal alliances with survivors is that it is the union, or at least, the public sector worker, who may represent the face of an oppressive mental health system. As much as survivors may wish to join forces and defend health and social care provision, their genesis as an alternate political force is fundamentally grounded in anger at the failings of welfare provision and bio-medical psychiatry – anger that is trenchant and justified.

In this light, trade unionists must not take it for granted that public services are popular – they may be regarded with scepticism or even hostility by the public and social movements alike. So, in pursuing reciprocal alliances between survivors and trade unions, unequal power dynamics have to be negotiated and must not be wished away by neoliberal gesturing in the direction of "consultation" and/or "empowerment." Of course, a complicating factor here, but one that also provides the groundwork for true reciprocity, is that workers may be members of "the system" – as trade union representatives, for instance – but, also, simultaneously, as fellow survivors, families, and friends.

Survivor movements, then, not only make demands upon the welfare state, they seek a transformed and emancipatory mental health system. More than this, they also aspire to a transformation of the power relations pervading our everyday lives. This latter observation provides a key to understanding the curious dynamic noted in our examples above, concerning the fraught relationships between survivors and workers after the lengthy Sheffield strike. Survivors, having tasted power and freedom through political activism, were no longer content to revert to the role of a passive recipient of welfare predicated, as such a role undoubtedly is, upon a distinction between them being labeled as "mad" and us (the workers) being legitimized as "mentally healthy." So, not only were survivors challenging an essential distinction between madness and sanity, but by extrapolation, they were also challenging a number of other fundamental dualisms – so taken for granted that we consider them "common sense" – upon which our Western culture and our public institutions rest. Such dualisms include the apparently commonsense distinctions between health and illness, normality and abnormality, disability and able-bodiedness, the worthy and unworthy recipients of welfare, and the survivor/worker distinction itself.

The troubling of these dualisms means that, although reciprocal challenges are necessarily a two-way street, they remain, nonetheless, asymmetrical. The challenge posed by the organized labour movement to the survivor movement has perhaps been the less well articulated of the two but involves the survivor movement engaging with the challenges faced by mental health workers within the constraints of the neoliberal project and a bio psychiatric frame-work. Yet, the two-way street is asymmetrical precisely insofar as recognition of the justified anger of survivors represents a non-negotiable condition of possibility for trade unionists who seek a democratization of the mental health system. To put it in a nutshell: autonomous survivor movements can do without trade unionists; but trade unionists who seek a democratization of psychiatry can-not do without survivors. What we are suggesting here is that deeply engaged relationships between trade unionists and survivors neces-sarily entail a paradoxical questioning of the public service cultures within which union activists work and a paradoxical questioning of our roles and responsibilities as workers within (and survivors of) them.

One peril here is that such paradoxical questioning risks co-optation at the hands of neoliberalism, which seeks to claw back the gains of the welfare state under the ideological banner of "respon-sibility," "self-care," and "recovery." Examples of self-organization can all too readily be used as an excuse to reduce welfare services in the name of combating the so-called "welfare dependency" culture in the UK. Similarly, what may be reasonable challenges to the "expertise" of mental health workers can inadvertently be used as ammunition for attacking worker's autonomy, decision making, and collectivization – and it is precisely these conditions that are being undermined by successive governments in the UK. Yet it is these very attributes that have historically helped workers forge the important alliances we referred to earlier. It is also what has enabled workers to fight for welfare advances for individual survivors whilst pre-serving collective provision. These paradoxes are not easy to resolve but require serious consideration lest we fall into the dual trap of either merely "defending the welfare state" or being lock, stock, and barrel "against" the mental health system in a way that may be counterproductive.

In these debates we often turn back to Peter Sedgwick whose lifework provides a number of lessons which, whilst requiring re-articulation today (see Cresswell and Spandler 2009), helps us plot a path through these paradoxes. We need to defend the welfare state against the encroachments of the neoliberal project because it is only within the context of State-funded welfare systems that the needs of human beings in distress can be met *en masse* in a complex modern society. But this observation invokes possibilities and perils all of its own. One peril is the political defensiveness of trade unions that may, understandably, respond to crises of the neoliberal project ("austerity" measures) by a reactionary defense of jobs and conditions to the exclusion of everything else. The problem here, as Sedgwick observed, is that the political analyses that underpin such a reaction are predicated upon economism, or what used to be referred to, pejoratively, as "vulgar" Marxism.

Such a negation is not just dualistically about us (workers) and them (e.g. those labeled "mad"). Rather, it attempts to subsume both identities beneath the collective pronoun we (Brown 1995). In advancing the cause of the welfare state on the grounds that it provides for the mass provision of welfare, any alliance, by necessity, defends the public sector against the twin encroachments of the neoliberal project: privatization and marketization. Therefore, our point of departure remains the imperative for political activism and the advance and transformation of the welfare state. Any minimal-Statism or welfare contractualism à la Hayek (2001), Popper (1945), or Szasz (1977) remain, therefore, deeply problematic.

Yet, the primacy that we accord the public sector inevitably raises another question about the role and value of the voluntary sector. Indeed, the other dualism that we want to problematize is that between the "public" and the "voluntary" sectors themselves. It is because we recognize the need to transform everyday life and not just the political economy of welfare provision that we require both thriving public *and* voluntary sectors. Indeed, it is perhaps because the voluntary sector lies outside "the bureaucratic compass of the State" that it is more able to promote the sorts of radical innovations that answer some of the transformative demands of survivors (Sedgwick 1982, 252). This means that seeing every form of alternative provision merely as a form of "privatization," as some trade union activists do, is equally problematic.

Furthermore, we need to be as concerned with the personal as well as the political aspects of activism. This requires being animated by the lessons of feminism and engaging with feminist critiques of both trade union organizing and survivor movement politics (Lewis 2007). Trade union alliances with survivors, notwithstanding that they are, of course, properly Political with a capital "P," are simultaneously personal with a lower case "p." Deeply engaged relationships between survivors and workers may threaten us, may challenge us, and may throw into disturbing relief what Pierre Bourdieu (1990) has called our habitus: our most deeply defended political and personal beliefs. But this particular peril – which can feel itself like a form of madness – is simultaneously a possibility that we may also strive to embrace. In other words, the asymmetrical reciprocity within survivor/worker alliances may be – and indeed, should be – unsettling for all participants (Church 1995). In this context it is vital to consider the importance of various communicative spaces in which alliances – however imperfect and unsettling they may be – can develop and flourish.

COMMUNICATIVE SPACES

Without the space for dialogue and reciprocity, political alliances will be superficial and are likely to flounder at the first hurdle. Elsewhere, we have pointed to the value of both "convergent spaces," which bring together reciprocal interests, and also "paradoxical" spaces, where issues of difference and diversity may be explicitly addressed (Spandler 2006, 2009). Here it is the very interaction of different perspectives that makes room for the creative imaginings of alternatives. Habermas's (1986, 1987) theory of communicative action suggests one way in which we might think about the quality and the asymmetry of relationships between survivor and worker activists and how it might be possible to piece together an alternative politics of mental health in democratic dialogue (McKeown 2012). Following Habermas, an ideal type of communication within an alliance could be framed in terms of deliberative democracy, wherein all participants are respectful of difference, power imbalances are acknowledged and reduced, and each participant attempts a presentation of arguments whilst remaining open to persuasion by the other's point of view.

Such a communicative space need not privilege a narrow conception of Western reason – as Fyodor Dostoevsky[8] once remarked, where human experience is concerned, 2 + 2 sometimes equals 5 – but would give equal weight to the expression of emotion, generally, and rage specifically. This form of democratic reciprocity will undoubtedly be difficult to achieve in the first instance and will inevitably be a "work in progress." Although critical survivor academics such as Peter Beresford (2010) and others (Barnes et al. 2007) have argued that deliberative structures may be one way of democratizing user involvement practices, Hodge (2005, 2009) points out that current communicative spaces fall a long way short of Habermasian ideals. But communicative spaces involving survivors and workers in alliance would aspire to represent a radically different order of dialogue than the typically "reasonable" formats beloved of top-down strategies of "user involvement."

More tellingly, other critics have called into question the value of communicative action in a mental health context. Primarily, this boils down to finding fault with the notion of "rationality" or "reasonableness" at the heart of the Habermasian theory. A number of problems arise from this concept, the most obvious being the extent to which survivor voices have historically been subjugated or silenced on the grounds of their putative irrationality (Bracken and Thomas 2005, Campbell 2009, Coleman 2008). The criticism also extends to a perceived neglect of important aspects of communication such as emotions and non-verbal expressiveness and psychological theories, which rely upon a prejudicial account of "disordered communication" (Barnes 2008, Crossley 2004). Not wishing to throw the rationalist baby out with the bathwater, Gardiner (2004) makes a case for revising the theory to take account of this critique whilst keeping hold of the central idea of reasoned deliberative democracy and its usefulness for disability movement activism.[9] But this is insufficient in the context of survivor/worker alliances, as we point out above, because deliberative democracy in the context of such alliances must acknowledge both the principle of asymmetrical reciprocity and a wider definition of "reason" that incorporates survivor experience and knowledge. After all, the survivor movement has a noble history of its own in providing a persuasive, reasoned, and moral critique of bio-psychiatry and an equally compelling vision for change. These kinds of discussions, debates, and alliances are happening in various contexts internationally. To give one example from the UK, they are promoted in the pages of *Asylum: The Magazine for Democratic Psychiatry*.[10]

CONCLUSIONS: RECIPROCAL ALLIANCES BECAUSE "ANOTHER WORLD IS POSSIBLE"

We have made a case for the development of progressive alliances between survivors and workers as one means of challenging and transforming the limitations of the mental health system. Whilst replete with a number of "perils and possibilities," we have suggested that reciprocal democratic relations can open up the possibilities for reframing the politics of mental health in ways that escape the strictures of narrow bio-medical psychiatry and the paradoxes of state-provided healthcare. If the possibilities we argue for are to transcend the perils we outline, then a number of key factors are germane from our reading of previous attempts at alliance formation.

These include the communicative spaces in which alliances are formed, and the extent to which they offer the sort of democratic space within which equal and imaginative reciprocity can emerge. These alliances offer a glimpse or "prefiguration" of the different kinds of social relations that we seek in a transformed society. Overlain on this is the quality of any media coverage, and the need to offer a concerted challenge to narratives that might undermine solidarity. The presence of politicized individual survivors and workers who can take the first steps to extend the hand of reciprocity and subsequently work hard to sustain the alliance is important on both sides of the relationship. However, the heaviest burden of responsibility for initiating these relationships will be placed on workers – that is precisely what we mean by asymmetrical reciprocity. In addition, reciprocity cannot be taken for granted just because a simplistic reason for a common cause can be located – asymmetrical reciprocity will be the enemy of alliance formation if it is not made the point of departure for democratic dialogue. Lastly, if reciprocity is easier to forge *against* something, rather than *for* something else, then building communicative spaces for dialogue is necessary sooner rather than later.

Trade unions and survivor groups clearly face significant challenges if they are to establish the sort of alliances we envisage here. Yet we remain hopeful. There are grounds for the sort of optimism that finds possibilities even in perils and, ultimately, views recalcitrance and resistance in the face of neoliberalism and bio-medical psychiatry as essentially creative acts. One person's peril, after all, is another's possibility.

NOTES

1 C. Millon-Delsol, "Barbarity and Solidarity," *Znak* 543 (2000): 51–9. http://tischner.org.pl/thinking_pliki/thinking_1/tischner_6_delsol.pdf. Last accessed 30 August 2012.
2 NALGO – the National Association of Local Government Officers, later to be merged into UNISON in 1992.

3 A. Roberts, "Scotland the Brave," *Mental Health Today* (July/August 2009). http://studymore.org.uk/mhtscot.htm. Last accessed 9 November 2012.
4 Ibid.
5 Millon-Delsol, "Barbarity and Solidarity," 51–9.
6 A good example can be found in: A. Plumb, "Incorporation, or Not, of MH Survivors into the Disability Movement" (paper presented at Distress or Disability? Proceedings from a symposium held at Lancaster University 15–16 November 2011). http://www.lancs.ac.uk/cedr/publications/Anderson_Sapey_and_Spandler_eds_2012.pdf. Last accessed 9 November 2012.
7 "Relational Organising: A Practical Guide for Trade Unionists," L. O'Halloran, 2006. www.newunionism.net/.../organizing/O'Halloran. Last accessed 5 January 2012.
8 See *Notes from the Underground* (1864).
9 See also the work of Iris Young who makes the case for less exclusionary deliberation. For example, I. Young, "Difference as a resource for democratic communication," in *Deliberative Democracy: Essays on Reason and Politics*, eds J. Bohman and W. Rehg, 383–406. Cambridge: MIT Press, 1997.
10 *Asylum: The Magazine for Democratic Psychiatry*, Special Issue: Anti Capitalism and Mental Health 19, no. 3 (2012). http://www.asylumonline.net/portfolio/19-3-autumn-2012/. Last accessed 9 November 2012.

11

Trans Jeopardy / Trans Resistance: Shaindl Diamond (SD) Interviews Ambrose Kirby (AK)

This is an interview that took place between Shaindl Diamond and Ambrose Kirby in Toronto, Ontario in September 2012. Both are locally involved in organizing resistance to psychiatry as activists and psychotherapists.

SD: Can you tell me a bit about your experience as a trans person vis-à-vis psychiatry and the kinds of problems that you've seen in the psychiatric system for trans people?

AK: What I see happening within trans[1] communities is a real effort to get our identities out of the DSM – out of a pathologizing framework. There has been an increasing willingness by health centres and individual health providers across Canada to recognize trans identity as regular, normal, not pathological. However, while our identities are being normalized, our resistance to transphobia is increasingly being separated out from our identities and pathologized. Instead of being trans people who creatively survive transphobia, we are trans people with anxiety disorders, anger disorders, bipolar [disorder], schizophrenia. Our basic identities are less and less considered a "mental illness," but our strategies for surviving are being taken out of context and individualized as "mental illnesses." So that, to me, is the big shift that I see happening.

In the last two years, I've been working at the Sherbourne Health Centre as a trans programs coordinator, working with trans youth and adults who are considering transition or are in the process of transition.[2] In this work, I receive calls from people all over the province and outside the province too. In all of that work,

the thing that stuck with me the most is the degree to which people are caught up in the psychiatric system. For most trans people
in Ontario, the only way to access transition is by going through
a lengthy process at the Centre for Addiction and Mental Health
(C A M H)[3] – many are forced to travel or move so they can get a
psychiatric label that will get them access to basic health care. If
there are services where they live, most people will still have to be
assessed by a psychiatrist and get a label. And no matter what, if
you want access to government-funded surgeries, you have to go
through C A M H. On top of that, an alarming number of both
adults and youth have additional psychiatric labels like depression, anxiety, bipolar, O C D, and A D D.

Increasingly too, I find that people, particularly youth, are seeking out a psychiatric label. There's a whole, insidious process here.
There's the desire to be validated for the struggle that they've gone
through, and there's financial struggles that are sometimes insur-
mountable. A lot of trans people are struggling at the edge of poverty. Some go into sex work voluntarily or involuntarily, and
increasingly people apply for the Ontario Disability Support Plan
(O D S P).[4] The way to access O D S P support for many trans people
is to agree that "I have a mental illness" beyond gender issues.
O D S P is a more viable option for youth and especially older folks
faced with huge financial barriers. Sex work can be a viable option
for trans people too. It's good money, you don't have to have
proper I D, you can assert who you are and be respected in your
chosen gender identity. Yet, it's also fraught with all kinds of danger, criminalization, harassment, and isolation. So when you can't
get work because of transphobia or a gendered work history, those
two options can feel like the only viable ones for people. So,
there's the legitimacy part, and there's the financial part.

Recently, at the Rainbow Health Ontario (R H O) Conference in
Ottawa, the psychologist and psychiatrist that run the gender
clinic for adults at C A M H did a presentation on what they call a
new approach to the recently re-released Standards of Care[5] for
trans people. They gave examples of when they would block someone from transitioning – they didn't call it "block" but that's what
it is – and one of the examples was: when someone had struggled
with anxiety, and really struggled to leave their house and got a
family member to do most of the things that they needed to do
outside of the house so that they wouldn't have to leave the house.

This is an example of someone they would try to block from transitioning until they got their so-called "anxiety" under control. Another example I heard was someone who's suicidal, really desperately wants to transition but can't because they're depending on CAMH, and CAMH is saying, "Until you have one year when you haven't tried to kill yourself, we won't consider allowing you to have surgery." The implications of that are astounding.

SD: So it's like they're treating gender identity as totally discrete from all these other kinds of struggles people have.

AK: Yes. Exactly. As though you're not anxious to leave the house because you're trans. It's just a thing you have. It's a "mental illness" that struck you inexplicably. Not really sure why.

A person I know was told they had a so-called "psychiatric problem" and recently, after years of being on lithium, they came out to their psychiatrist as trans. The psychiatrist was like, "Oh, OK, well let me re-look at what this diagnosis is." Like, suddenly they don't have a "mental illness," you know?

SD: So you mean, all that other stuff got erased in favour of gender identity disorder in that psychiatrist's eyes?

AK: Yeah – anything can be anything, if the psychiatrist says it is. So, you know, you can have schizophrenia, which they insist is genetic or actually "Oops! No, you're just trans." Clearly there's no illness involved.

SD: It sounds like, from what you're saying, the gender identity disorder diagnosis is, in itself, not being conceptualized as illness in the same way.

AK: No, it is. But that's changing. The same way that the lesbian, gay, bisexual community mobilized to remove those identities from the DSM, similar actions are happening around trans identity.[6] So, it's not that psychiatrists don't think it's an illness, it's that the trans community doesn't think it's an illness, and increasingly medical and health care professionals are getting on board and recognizing that, including the World Professional Association for Trans Health (WPATH).[7]

CAMH has gone through some changes, including hiring people who were considered allies within the trans community to do the approvals. So, on the surface, there seemed to be positive changes. But in fact, these allies have really maintained the status quo, just with new language. So, when the new WPATH standards of care came out in September 2011, shortly thereafter a bulletin was

issued by C A M H about how they planned to integrate these exciting changes. When I was at W P A T H in September, when they
announced the re-modeled Standards of Care, one of the very first
things that was said by the committee representative who was presenting the changes was: "There. Are. No. More. Real-life. Tests."
And people were ecstatic. They were so excited about it. So when
C A M H put out their "changes" they accepted to have no more
real-life tests. Instead, there's going to be "The Gender Role
Experience."

S D : How long is that for?

A K : It's twelve months, and it's the same criteria. According to
them, you can start hormones after three months. But there's still a
year-long waiting list to get in. There are still several appointments
that you have to go through first before they can say "Yes, you can
start hormones." They've changed the questionnaire because that
was a big stumbling block for a lot of people. They've eliminated
all the questions except for personal info and one question: "Tell us
your life story." But in fact, they now just include questions like
"what do you fantasize about while you masturbate" in the interview instead. At that conference that I already mentioned, the
Rainbow Health Ontario (R H O) Conference in Ottawa, I asked
the C A M H people directly about that. I asked why that was necessary. And it was very clear that they think it's an important and relevant question to ask somebody in addition to how often they
masturbate and what their sexual orientation is. Myself and
another activist and psychotherapist asked those very direct questions, and they defended their right to know saying that these are
relevant and important answers to get before allowing somebody
to transition.

For sure, some changes have happened as a result of community
pressure. But the point is that people are still being directed to go
through the hoops of psychiatrists to get access to medical transition. And it's clear that psychiatry is holding onto the right to classify and determine the best course of action for us. There is
movement outside of C A M H, within medical and healthcare circles, to shift more towards an "informed consent" model. This
would mean that adults, above eighteen, who are making decisions about their life and their bodies, as long as they are being
informed in a thorough way about the risks and consequences

attending transition, have the right to choose. I mean, it's so basic, but to the gender clinics and psychiatry, the informed consent model doesn't make sense. They are content to keep themselves as gatekeepers.

The effects of transphobia in trans people's lives – and of course all the other violent experiences they have with structures of power like race, class, and ability – are so profound. I mean, trans people are among the poorest groups. Poverty is through the roof. People can't get housing or well-paying, secure jobs despite being a highly educated population.[8] Because of the effects of all of that, people need to turn somewhere for support and because of this rampant discourse of mental health and mental illness, the only place to turn, for a large part, is either psychiatry or people who are working from deeply within a psychiatric model.

So people are still turning to CAMH for transition. Fortunately, there are now more people outside of CAMH willing to work to create access for trans people. What CAMH does, in terms of pressuring trans people to jump through so many hoops that are quite abusive, is looked down upon by people outside of CAMH in pretty dignified ways. At the same time most folks who are critical of CAMH for how they deal with medical transition are still very committed to the erroneous idea that there is such a thing as mental illness. People who are otherwise quite progressive – in terms of defending their bodies and their right to access and their right not to have to go to CAMH and their right not to be seen as mentally ill simply because they're trans – are still committed to the idea that mental illness does exist, just not in me or just not because I'm trans, but because my mom had it or because it's genetic or it's in my family or because that's the way I am. People are really up in arms about not having to be labeled as mentally ill because they are trans. However, they're very much still committed to the possibility that you can be trans and have a mental illness.

SD: But in terms of the transitioning piece itself, would you say that people are turning more to other avenues outside of CAMH to get support around transitioning?

AK: Yes. Yes, but it's still really slim. Like, in Toronto, it's pretty much a couple of health centres, with a few doctors in private practice too. There are a few other health centres, like in Guelph, Windsor, Thunder Bay, and Ottawa. So there are places across

Ontario that are actively working to support trans people with transition. What that means, technically, is getting access to hormones, and information, and community sometimes as well. It doesn't mean surgery. Still, to get access to O H I P -funded surgeries, you have to go through C A M H .

s d : With the new Standards of Care and these kinds of new directions being put out there, do you see that changing? Even if the change is not giving total power to trans people themselves to make decisions about their bodies, is there a shift to put that power in the hands of other types of health care professionals or other doctors outside of the C A M H clinic?

a k : Well, what's exciting about the new W P A T H standards of care is they explicitly state that in order to get approved for surgery, people need the support of two medical or healthcare professionals who are competent in this field. The wording is really particular in that regard. It doesn't say anywhere that those healthcare professionals need to be psychiatrists. The qualification is that you need a Master's degree and some competency and experience working with trans people. That's it. So, nowhere does it say that you have to jump through the hoops of psychiatry and answer questions about your sexual fantasies and how you masturbate – that's C A M H holding onto its old gate-keeping, oppressive ways.

Practically, getting psychiatry to relinquish control over trans people's lives is very hard. It's probably a big long fight. And whether we ever succeed in getting totally outside of psychiatry, I don't know. What's happened in the last five years is there was a huge effort to get a couple more sites that would be recognized by O H I P, outside of C A M H . It was a good three or four years of work. It was a high-level negotiation. It was report writing and paperwork and stats and long meetings and dialogue and negotiation with C A M H . At the end of the day, what happened is there wasn't a political will in government to make that change.

s d : You spoke about adults and this idea that adults can make important decisions about transitioning and changes they want to go through medically. Have you any thoughts about children? How do children fit into that picture?

a k : I do. I think kids are not respected enough. Children know exactly what they need. By that, I don't mean they know if they're trans or not, but they know that "wearing this shirt feels bad" or "I get so excited to play with this toy." All we need to do is follow their lead about what empowers them. Children are so revealing in that way. You can see in an instant whether something is working or not for them. I think we need only to follow that lead and not make decisions. We don't need to know if they're just different, just trans, just gay, just whatever. Children will tell you when they're ready. For sure by puberty or teenage-hood, youth really begin to be able to articulate more and more who they are and make some decisions with support. Support is key, support for parents to be able to tolerate that their children might know something that they can't possibly begin to understand. I think, more than anything, children need to be protected from getting diagnosed.

People do have big problems in living, but I fundamentally believe that the medical model, the psychiatric pathological model of human behavior, is scientifically unfounded and is unhelpful in terms of getting at the heart of what human beings need to thrive. And children are especially vulnerable to that. It can happen in a few different ways. Really loving parents turn to authorities that they expect to have some kind of knowledge or wisdom and get sucked in. Or, there are people who want to fix their children and make sure that they don't turn out gay or trans and so they take them to people like [Ken] Zucker at CAMH and he helps them with that. He doesn't help the children; he helps the parents stay stuck and keeps the children disenfranchised.

And then there's just neglect. A lot of the youth that I work with have such intense histories of trauma and violence, sexual abuse, neglect, intense poverty, parents who provide neither food nor nurturing. Some children get kicked out or told they're bad because they're different or they get humiliated routinely by teachers and students at school because they're different. So, the trauma of not fitting in and the violence that comes with that, this is what is happening to youth. Their social awkwardness is getting labeled, their anger is getting labeled, their cutting and self-harm is getting labeled, their extreme rage when they're pushed is getting labeled. Yet, no one wants to talk about the abuse that children go through, the complete disempowerment that they face, and the disbelief that can be so damaging.

sd: Do you think we can create services that meet the needs of trans people within psychiatric institutions?

ak: As long as we, as trans people or gender different people, continue to subscribe to the psychiatric model in any regard, we put ourselves at risk, and we put other people at risk. It's not enough to get our identities out of the DSM, because somebody else's identity is in there. It doesn't say in the DSM anywhere "young, black men's anger syndrome," but it might as well. There are a disproportionate number of young black men diagnosed with schizophrenia. Soon it may not say "gender identity disorder," but it will say "anger disorders," "oppositional defiance disorder," "anxiety disorder." They might as well call those "people who have been oppressed disorders." And that includes us as trans people. So, it's not enough to just take our identities out of the DSM, and it's not enough to have this psychiatric model that we tweak. It's a model that we need to get rid of, and we need to get rid of it precisely because, at the heart of that model is this idea of mental illness – mental illness that you cannot find in the brain if you do an autopsy.

Let me put that into context. One of the people who is writing the new version of the diagnosis for "gender dysphoria" for children is Zucker at CAMH. He has been widely discredited for his views that children who are cross-gender identifying or who are gender independent can be "cured" through reparative therapy. "They were assigned female at birth? No problem! We'll make sure they turn into a good little girl. Here's what you do: Deny them the opportunity to hang out with boys, don't let them have so-called 'boy's toys.'" This is Ken Zucker's approach to gender independent children. And he's unabashedly unashamed about it. He is writing the pathological definition of what it means to be a gender creative kid and how to fix it. He's the "expert" who is majorly contributing to this section of the DSM.

This whole structure is so obviously flawed that if we simply take ourselves out of the DSM or out of CAMH and go to the psychiatrists at the Sherbourne Health Centre or Hincks-Dellcrest[9] to get our support and approvals, we will continue to be pathologized. What we'll do is we'll become complicit in erasing the context of our own and other people's struggle for self-determination.

SD: That makes a lot of sense in terms of theoretically where things have been headed and practical implications for that. I am wondering about when pockets of alternative programming are created within the system.

AK: Are you thinking about the Hincks-Dellcrest?

SD: Yeah, I was thinking about that. You know, at the Gender and Sexual Orientation Service at the Hincks-Dellcrest, children don't go there to get diagnoses. But it's still within this institution, and there's a gatekeeper. It's just a gatekeeper with a different vision.

A K : It's not enough. As long as we're talking about mental health, we're not talking about solidarity, support, community development, access. That's what we're actually talking about. So people who are setting themselves up as gatekeepers or insisting that people who are gender-different or gender-independent need to go to clinics to get support, are missing a huge part of the puzzle, which is the social, the societal – a political issue that prevents adults and children from being who they are.

Discourses around disability are really amazing at identifying what the real problem is – the barriers presented by a society that refuses to acknowledge that it's through power that we erase people and prevent them from getting access to society. Let me say that a different way because I said "we" and it assumes that people with disabilities aren't part of the "we." That's the problem; the "we" is the normative, the dominant group, and everyone outside is seen as imposing on the norm to get special access. Whereas, gender-independent kids are everywhere, kids with disabilities are everywhere, adults with disabilities are everywhere. All kinds of people with all kinds of variations and differences and uniqueness are everywhere. That is actually what society means; it's everyone.

S D : What is your vision for how you would like to see the trans community move forward in terms of activism and initiatives?

A K : I see many possible directions. This year, the title of the Canadian Professional Association for Trans Health (C P A T H) conference is "Beyond Pathology." So, there's an awareness that we need to get trans people outside of this pathologized model and integrated in a more meaningful way into all aspects of life – and not just included as an add-on to professional knowledge about healthcare or education or prison. And I like that shift. I like it because the Trans Pulse Survey that surveyed about 500 trans people living in Ontario came out with the result that almost 75% of trans people had either attempted suicide or actively considered it. Seventy-five percent! And that's the ones who are still alive, never mind all the people who have killed themselves. The other thing that they found is that suicide risk is the highest at the very point when someone has decided to transition and they get blocked from transition. That means C A M H 's one-year waiting list to get a first interview, that means being interrogated about sexual preferences, that means having gatekeepers tell you how long you have to prove to them that you've been "stable" before you can access hormones or surgery, that means not being able to go across town to your family doctor for info and access, never mind all the other hoops about changing your name. And how do you apply for a job when all of your work history is gendered or you can't get references from the past? There are so many hoops right there when people are at the point of wanting to take a risk to really be themselves. So I think that's where I see the activism happening; in that zone; creating quicker, 'informed-consent access' to transition and beyond – access to schooling, work, housing, all of those kinds of basic things.

I feel that same fear about psychiatry as I do about the prison industrial complex and trans people; that there's this intense risk of being erased as a person, a creative person who has survived. I don't know how to describe it, but usually I describe it as, before transition, I was under the surface of life, and after transition, I'm able to break that surface and see what's out there in life. Of course, not all trans people are going to identify in that way, or want to transition, or all of those things.

I'm trying to make this a bit personal as well and say I don't know what the big picture answers are. I see little pieces about de-pathologizing trans people, but also de-pathologizing our resistance to transphobia. That's the key and that's going to happen in so many different ways, through art and culture, through politics and through education and healthcare, the whole works, housing, shelter. People are doing amazing things out there in different ways.

s d : Do you see people in the trans community working in antipsychiatry or psychiatric survivor initiatives? Do you see much crossover, or areas where there could be crossover where there isn't?

a k : Well, in terms of psychiatric survivor organizing, a crossover I see is around access to supportive health care services, not pathologizing ones. Trans people do need access to medical procedures, medical hormones, surgery, and often want to have supportive counselling services, not because there's something inherently wrong with us and we need to sort it out in counselling, but because we face so much oppression. You know, there's so much stigma and shame. We are communities that are shunned by society as a rule. If you experience other realities, if you are assigned "male" at birth and you wear a dress; these are equivalent in our society to being unacceptable: "there's something wrong with you." The most benevolence we can hope for is "It's not your fault that you are like this or that this happened to you." So, in terms of resisting that individual pathologization, there's so much overlap between being trans and being a psychiatric survivor.

In terms of antipsychiatry organizing, I can't think of a community that is better suited to take part than the trans community – except for the fatigue in terms of having to struggle day in and day out to walk down the street, to talk on the phone, to have a job, to sit in school, to be in public. Aside from the fatigue factor, working to abolish psychiatry and abolish prisons would do wonders for trans people. It would eliminate two options by which we are routinely dismissed and discredited. And it would force people to have to deal with our difference and the fact that trans people are under-housed, over-drugged, too visible yet invisible, and marginal. So I see a lot of potential for alliances and combined actions between all of those communities.

s d : Do you see any barriers? I know you spoke about how tiring it is to experience oppression in many different ways, on a daily basis. That can really make it hard for people to engage in some manifestations of political action. Are there any other kinds of barriers preventing that from happening?

a k : I think trans people are working tirelessly to get out from the DSM in such a way that it could lead to distancing ourselves from those who have been psychiatrized, even though we are people who are psychiatrized. A common stance is "I'm not disabled," "I'm not mentally ill," which is not helpful because there are people who identify as being disabled, and they don't feel that that's a curse word or lesser identity, and they shouldn't. And I know that there are other trans people who identify as disabled or as psychiatric survivors so there's already overlap that's happening. Eli Clare[10] is coming to mind. But I think, just as any other community, we're very much caught up in dominant narratives about who's normal and who's not. And we've definitely internalized a lot of that. "Who passes" is a big one in our community. Who's a real trans person, who isn't? Gender non-conforming or gender-queer people are not considered trans enough sometimes. There's as much difference in our communities as there is in any community, and that can pose barriers to solidarity. Competing for scarce resources is always a barrier. It is classic divide-and-conquer. If we're always competing with each other then we're fighting ourselves instead of working with other communities to make broader social change.

I don't think in antipsychiatry or psychiatric survivor circles there is a lot of awareness about what happens to trans people in psychiatry. I haven't seen that. I don't want to make huge generalizations, but in my experience, it hasn't been very important.

A very interesting barrier that I face is that I'm dependent on CAMH to approve me for surgery. I'm really stuck at the moment. I'm so angry that I can't even make myself put pen to paper and fill out that application. As an anti-psychiatry activist, to willingly submit myself to CAMH for examination and approval feels so mind-blowingly terrible. It's a huge barrier for me. It makes sense that people don't want to fight psychiatry because we're dependent on them. That's huge. I've had the application for six months. It's just sitting there.

SD: That's really hard.

AK: It's so hard. So, the daily dependence on psychiatry precludes the possibility of organizing against psychiatry in some pretty major ways. That goes for not only accessing surgery, but accessing financial supports as I said.

SD: Is there anything you want to add?

AK: Yeah. As a white, trans man, a lot of what I'm saying is loaded with my own perspective and my own identity. I haven't meaningfully addressed status issues, immigration issues, prisoner issues. But I wanted to speak, to try in my way to contribute to this conversation. I hope that this will be, at some point, one of many voices talking about this from different perspectives.

I don't have all the technical inside and out knowledge, but I do know that trans people are disproportionately told that there's something wrong with us. And most of us end up in a relationship with psychiatry. Whenever the numbers are that high, there's something to be extremely concerned about. Indigenous youth are experiencing suicide or thinking that that's a viable option in staggering numbers in this country – the same goes with trans youth and adults. That suicide is such a viable option is not just sad or tragic; it's a sign of a bigger political and social problem. Like indigenous youth, trans people aren't born wanting to die – we live in a world that actively resists our existence and seeks to control and contain us. We don't need psychiatry, we need solidarity and justice. We need room to live.

S D : Thank you, Ambrose.

NOTES

1 Trans refers here to a range of identities including but not limited to transsexual, transgender, gender queer, gender independent, M T F, F T M, M T M, F T F, transgirl, transboi, transman, and transwoman. It is still an insufficient term to represent the stories and diversity of all people who identify in these ways. We use it to begin a conversation, not to limit or contain it.

2 I do not represent the Sherbourne Health Centre in any way. I name it because it was there, in contact with so many trans people, that I really saw the depth of trans people's involvement in psychiatry.

3 C A M H is the Centre for Addiction and Mental Health, a psychiatric institution in Toronto, with a long history of violence against trans people. It is the only assessment site for government funded trans-related surgeries for Ontario, Newfoundland, and Manitoba, and is a main referral site for a majority of trans people seeking to transition medically.

4 O D S P is the Ontario Disability Support Plan. A person on O D S P can expect to have a monthly income that is a few hundred dollars more than the amount of regular social assistance.

5 The Standards of Care (S O C) for trans people were initially developed by sexologist Harry Benjamin. Currently, the World Professional Association for Trans Health (W P A T H) produces the S O C. Version 7, released in 2012, can be found here: http://wpath.org/publications_standards.cfm

6 However, I would like to stress that despite these efforts, homosexuality continued to appear in the D S M as a disorder, whether it be called "ego-dystonic homosexuality" or other things. For a discussion of this phenomenon, see Burstow 1990.

7 Note the change in title, for example, between the W P A T H standards of care version 6: "Standards of Care for Gender Identity Disorders" and the new version 7: "Standards of Care for the Health of Transsexual, Transgender, and Gender Non-conforming People" (http://wpath.org/publications_standards.cfm).

8 See the Trans Pulse Project e-bulletins at http://transpulseproject.ca/research-type/e-bulletin/ for statistics relating to trans people in Ontario.

9 The Sherbourne Health Centre is a centre for trans-positive primary health care and social/educational supports for trans and gender creative people. The Hincks-Dellcrest is a centre for children and youth in Toronto and has a Gender and Sexual Identity Team.

10 "Eli Clare weaves hope, critical analysis, and compassionate storytelling together in his work on disability and queerness, insisting on the twine of race, class, gender, sexuality, and disability." See "Eli Clare: Writer, Speaker, Activist, Teacher, Poet," http://eliclare.com. Last accessed November 4, 2012.

12

Take it Public:
Use Art to Make Healing
a Public Narrative

ROSEMARY BARNES AND SUSAN SCHELLENBERG

INTRODUCTION

SUSAN: When my analysis work was coming to an end in 2003, I dreamed the face of a woman patient from 1953, my first year of nursing training. I was taught that the woman's rapidly clenching and unclenching over-bite jaw, foul language, chloral-hydrate[1] breath, and rage were signs that she suffered from a psychiatric condition diagnosed as Korsakoff's psychosis. The woman's presentation made it difficult for nurses to empathize with or go near her and, according to my dream, difficult for this nurse to forget her. I understood the dream to signal that this patient's plight was one of the true faces of sexual abuse that my culture had not previously recognized. I took the dream to confirm as well that the same patient's fate might have been mine had I not found ways to access and clear the traumatic core of my 1969 breakdown.

In 1969 as a young suburban mother of four small children, my three-week admission to Lakeshore Psychiatric Hospital began. On hospital discharge, my husband and I understood my diagnosis was schizophrenia. Convinced by my children's need of a well mother and by the definition of schizophrenia I learned as a nurse, I willingly submitted to taking prescribed anti-psychotic drugs. Motherhood, religion, a corporate/traditional style of marriage, and a view of my illness that conformed with society's "doctor/god/patient/victim" narrative discouraged my questioning why prescribed drugs were my only treatment. Until, after ten years, I came close to suicide under the care of a diagnosis and drug-focused psychiatric model. Soon after my decision to withdraw from drugs, I made deep commitments to heal my mind from the causes of my breakdown, to heal my body from the drug side effects, and to paint a record of my dreams as my mind and body healed. For some years, I studied art, gained more knowledge of dream interpretation, and painted regularly.

ROSEMARY: I trained as a clinical psychologist about seven years after Susan was hospitalized with a psychotic break. After postdoctoral training, I worked as staff psychologist at Toronto General Hospital, then chief psychologist at Women's College Hospital. I learned and practiced illness-focused, medical model care. I had a professional career that I understood and enjoyed until I realized that medical model care was often unhelpful and in some ways actually harmful to people seeking help. After trying and failing to reform hospital structures, I became lost and felt cynical, exhausted, and angry about my apparently successful career. I learned of Susan's experiences in 1992 when she exhibited her paintings at Women's College Hospital. What she had to say reflected much of what I found troubling.

SUSAN AND ROSEMARY: Since the 1990s, we have worked together as artist and psychologist to share what we have learned about healing from emotional pain[2] (see also Barnes and Schellenberg 2004, Schellenberg and Barnes 2009). We have never been in a doctor/patient relationship. In this chapter, we tell a little of our own stories and describe a postmodern perspective on resistance to medical model mental health care. We introduce "emotional pain" as words that hold open possibilities for naming and responding to experiences usually described publicly in medical model terms such as "mental illness" and "mental health care." We propose healing as an organizing narrative for emotional pain. We explain how public art events increase the visibility of ordinarily private stories where individuals with lived experience name and respond on their own terms rather than deferring to the words and constructs specified by mental health professionals. As private stories of healing are made public, they reduce the stigma attached to lived experience of the emotional pain usually known as "mental illness" and displace medical model care as the dominant societal narrative for naming and responding to emotional pain.

POSTMODERN THINKING ABOUT RESISTANCE AND CHANGE

ROSEMARY: As Susan and I talked and wrote about well being and healing (Barnes and Schellenberg 2004, Schellenberg and Barnes 2009), I came to appreciate the healing potential of public arts events. I was also interested in postmodern therapies and narrative therapy in particular (White and Epson 1991; Freedman and Combs 1996; White 2007, 2010). Arts events and postmodern approaches pointed out avenues for change that I had not considered.

Social discussion about individuals experiencing emotional pain often relies on a medical model narrative where the individual in distress is encouraged to see an expert doctor (i.e., physician, psychologist, social worker, and so on), and thus become a patient. The doctor asks about symptoms and provides a diagnosis, highlighting what is important and what meaning to ascribe to the patient's experiences. Typically, doctors diagnose patients as suffering from one of the mental illnesses listed in the American Psychiatric Association's diagnostic manual, the DSM-5 (American Psychiatric Association 2000, 2013). Patients are encouraged to return to normal by following the doctor's orders, e.g., take your medications or do the therapy homework. The experience is considered private.

The medical model approach is modern. A modern way of thinking assumes that "The truth is out there," i.e., that with enough study and effort, we can ascertain what is normal and what is illness. "Normal," "mental illness," and diagnoses are treated as referring to certainties or realities, not just ideas about how to understand life or emotional pain. A postmodern view, however, holds that reality is neither fixed nor certain, but instead constructed through attention and interpretation. Among the myriad possibilities of daily life, we notice or perceive some aspects of experience and ignore others. Through our ideas, talk, and practices, we organize perceptions into meanings, and meanings into narratives or stories. Beliefs about reality or "truth" develop from a continual process of noticing, deciding on meanings, and creating narratives. To keep life manageable, we adopt a few narratives as guides for what to notice and how to interpret what we notice. Such narratives can be described as dominant, and come to feel like reality. An individual's dominant narrative provides his or her primary basis for engaging in life. A society's dominant narratives provide the basis for social arrangements and practices, i.e., laws, policies, organizations, and resource allocation. For both individuals and societies, dominant narratives always co-exist with marginal or potential narratives – that is, unnoticed experiences that could be noticed and used to form meanings and stories, but that are not taken up and so remain peripheral in directing attention and action.

Illness-focused medical model care is a dominant social narrative. Such care has been critiqued for many years and for many reasons (see, for example, Bentall 1990; Bracken and Thomas 2005; Caplan 1995; Szasz 1974, 1988; Whitaker 2010). The most serious concern is that despite "advances" in care, outcomes for people identified as mentally ill are not better than they were sixty years ago and may well be worse (Whitaker 2010). Adoption of the medical model narrative does not ensure that those in emotional pain can expect to have better lives. Modernist defenders of the medical model argue that our understanding is imperfect, but that if we persist, if we do more and better-funded research, if we learn more about neurotransmitters, or genetics, or brain structure, then we will come closer and closer to the truth concerning mental illness and treatment. However, sixty years of such research has been largely unfruitful (Bentall 1990; Bracken and Thomas 2005; Szasz 1974, 1988; Whitaker 2010).

From a postmodern perspective, the central problem with the medical model narrative is not our imperfect understanding. The central problem is that the dominance of this narrative constricts individual and societal possibilities by encouraging the belief that mental illness is a fixed reality rather than just one among many possible ways of naming and responding to emotional pain (Raskin and Lewandowski 2000). Equating emotional pain to mental illness functions to suppress other possibilities, other meanings, and other stories for naming and responding to such pain. In order to explore other possibilities and to develop richer understandings of emotional pain and possible responses, postmodernists want to "discourage foreclosing meaning making experience through the preemptive adoption of only one construction of disorder" (Raskin and Lewandowski 2000, 19).

This well-known image (Figure 12.1) offers a visual illustration of what I have in mind. In this image, a black urn is present, but the

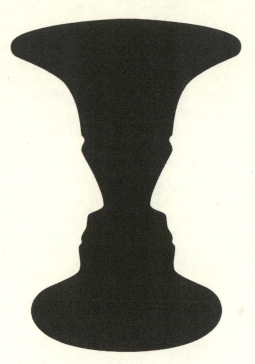

Figure 12.1   Urn/people visual image.
(Susan Schellenberg, *After Edgar Rubin's
Vase*. Reproduced with permission)

two people who appear to be conversing are also present. What is
reality? An individual's experience of the reality depends on the
individual's attentional focus at a given moment. Doctors conveyed
to Susan and her husband that Susan suffered from schizophrenia,
let's say an urn, so needed to be returned to her normal life as a wife
and mother. Susan, in the course of painting her dreams, identified
dialogues between her inner psyche and outer world awareness, that
provided new and deeply satisfying stories about herself and her life,
e.g., her wounded parents, her childhood pain, herself as an artist.
She attended to the people conversing. From a postmodern perspective, creating change has to do with directing attention. So, if we
prefer the story of people conversing rather than the story of the urn,
how can we direct attention to this story?

SUSAN: My dream art was first shown as part of Never Again, a
hospital event held to increase awareness about violence against

women.[3] The exhibit's art and text recorded my growth from my lowest point in 1980, after a ten-year course of anti-psychotic drugs, to the time of the exhibit. At journey's beginning, I was isolated in suburbia as well as psychologically and philosophically distanced from the survivor/anti-psychiatric movements. Where I now respect how the "my craziness is okay" response can be an essential coping tool for some, I could not adopt this option, as achieving a more whole sense of self through naming my "psychotic symptoms" as "normal and okay" was counter to my nursing training and my need as a mother to protect my own and my family's well being. Who I was then provided an ample supply of false selves for me to shed over the following years as I worked at creating a new self and life and at gaining the needed consciousness and psychic strength to resolve childhood trauma. The childhood trauma involved abuse experiences that I had deeply repressed and that prescribed anti-psychotic medication had further buried.

When my convent-school conditioning in ladylikeness collided with the near overpowering rage I developed during a four-year supervised withdrawal from anti-psychotic drugs, the anti-psychiatry literature of the time validated my rage but fell short of telling me how to make sense and let my rage go. Deep shame and concern for my children forced a dual role onto my rage, making it the foremost influence on my eventual commitments to become well and to keep an art and written record of my dreams and inner journey as my mind healed. Though I knew that my children would be affected by my psychosis and the ways that I was affected by anti-psychotic medication, I hoped that my art, writing, and commitment to healing would offer my family a lived story of healing whether or not they consciously chose to learn from it.

From the beginning, I followed a pattern where commitment preceded story, and story expression preceded growth in wellness. For example, one dream painting called *Bury it with Respect* (Figure 12.2) shows the head and shoulders of a bishop resting on leaves. In my dream, the bishop stood at the foot of my garden rockery and dissolved into a pile of dead leaves. Dream work led me to realize that the bishop's leaves signaled the difficult decisions to leave my marriage, religion, and home that I faced at that time while they were dually encouraging me to trust that those same leaving processes would fertilize and nourish my next stage of growth.

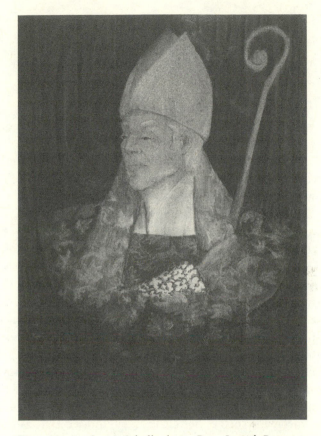

Figure 12.2   Susan Schellenberg, *Bury It with Respect*,
mixed media on paper, 27.5 x 38.25 inches. (Centre for
Addiction and Mental Health, Toronto. Reproduced
with permission)

Once I committed to heal and to record my dreams, mentors and
helpers bearing story, myth, art, drama, and movement skills began
to appear in my life. From that time onward each of my gains in
consciousness marked the slow dissolve of my rage. Each mentor
brought an aspect of story that allowed me to better see and express
my dream journey in art and later in writing. Art, dream, and story
helped me to recover, own, and resolve the story of my breakdown.
I came to regard healing as growth in ability to love and forgive
self and other, to cope, to feel pleasure, to engage in meaningful
activity, and to follow the psyche's inner direction away from

addiction and towards greater wholeness. This perspective is neither pro- nor anti-psychiatry.

EMOTIONAL PAIN

ROSEMARY: As Susan worked with her dreams and art, she identified a story of herself as abused, rageful, then healing. She preferred this story over the earlier story of herself as suffering from mental illness. In order to remain open to noticing preferred, but marginalized, stories of the kind that Susan tells, I began searching for words that are free of mental illness/medical model implications. I wanted to avoid medical model terminology unless in situations where I was discussing medical model constructs. A friend with lived experience suggested "emotional pain," and these words seemed right. I use "emotional pain" to describe difficulties that cause a person substantial distress, interfere with his or her ability to achieve important life goals, or interfere significantly with his or her ability to enjoy caring and mutually respectful relationships with others. I prefer "emotional pain" because these words are ordinary; are not associated with any theoretical or clinical construct; and are readily recognized as what individuals experience when life is not going well.

But emotional pain often feels frightening and chaotic. The medical model reassures because, despite its failings, it provides an organizing narrative for such experiences, both individually and socially. We need an organizing narrative for emotional pain. So, if not the medical model narrative, then what?

A NARRATIVE OF HEALING

Like most people living in emotional pain, Susan and I wanted to feel better in a sustainable way, that is, to heal in the way that Susan defines it above. Healing involves an improved sense of wellness and ability to engage in life, and is thus different from overcoming or curing a disease. Healing is always possible, even when cure is not. Healing requires committing to well-being and finding a refuge, then cultivating supportive relationships; an ecology of healing; and confidence in life's healing capacities (Schellenberg and Barnes 2009). What we describe as healing is similar to the recovery model (Davidson et al. 2005; Davidson, Harding, and Spaniol 2005a, 2005b; Jacobson 2004) chosen as a central focus for national mental health strategy by the Mental Health Commission of Canada.[4]

Susan's art relates a healing narrative. Such healing is not a rare exception, even among individuals diagnosed with serious mental illness. A wellness and healing-focused approach enables many people living with serious mental illness to make remarkable improvement or to recover (Davidson, Harding, and Spaniol 2005a, 2005b). But why should a private healing experience be presented publically?

SUSAN: By the mid-1990s, I had developed a collection of paintings that recorded my dreams as my mind and body healed. These works provided a psychological portrait of the emotional pain that doctors identified as a mental illness and demonstrated how dreams had guided and reflected the healing of my mind and body. When I read the work of art historian Suzi Gablick (1991), I became interested in art that is socially conscious and fosters interconnection. I was inspired by Gablick's view that an art aligned with other social disciplines could mirror the collective effort needed to save the planet as a place that sustains human life. As current human behaviours and systems threaten the earth's air, water, and living creatures, and thus human survival, I believe Gablick is right in arguing for art forms that embrace interdisciplinary collaboration and address the human spirit in ways that nurture its will to change.

After reading Gablick, I also began to recognize parallels between my own healing and the healing of the planet. Just as my painted dream images helped to knit together disparate fragments of myself to create a new life story, healing the planet can be helped through our knitting together disparate fragments of understanding to create a new story of ourselves and Great Mother Earth. I read Gablick close to the time I was invited to join my first multidisciplinary collaboration. From that time on, I began to realize that my own art could increase public awareness concerning the helpful role art and story can take in the healing and recovery process for an individual living in emotional pain and, by analogy, for a planet in pain.

My painting and involvement in socially engaged art at the 1992 Women's College Hospital Never Again event[5] led to an offer to fund a permanent exhibit of my dream paintings. Since the funding was conditional on the exhibit being mounted at a psychiatric teaching facility, I began discussions with the Centre for Addiction and

Mental Health (C A M H), a university-affiliated psychiatric hospital in Toronto. My mid-1990's collaboration with C A M H involved the permanent installation of my dream art and text in that facility's main lobby as the Shedding Skins exhibit. The decision to align my Shedding Skins art to a healing perspective meshed with my focus on healing from the early 1980s onward. Though able at the time to express myself visually and with the written word, I had yet to resolve the core issues of my breakdown, so at that time, lacked the clarity and awareness to articulate a broader focus. Hospital staff involved with the planning of the installation demonstrated unbiased, arm's length respect for my paintings and story through their careful listening and acknowledgement. Their stance encouraged me to proceed with the exhibit and to gain unexpected and significant healing from my exhibit involvement.

As my new vision of my life expanded, I better understood how the long-term daily ritual of taking psychoactive drugs had reinforced my and my husband's belief that psychiatry's initial illness diagnosis and treatment was justified. When that belief fused with the stigma of mental illness, it became near impossible to overcome. It is difficult now to believe that I ever held such harmful beliefs, let alone carried them forward until the mid-1990s. On completion of a series of conversations undertaken in preparation for the Shedding Skins installation and later for the Committed to the Sane Asylum book, these beliefs dissolved to the degree I was able to decline C A M H's offer to be named that year's "Courage to Come Back" award recipient. By then I knew that such an award would require me to play the role of a psychiatrically helped and saved patient and require me as well to deny both my wrongful psychiatric treatment and the new story that my art and writing on the book was uncovering.

Since its 1998 installation, Shedding Skins has been viewed by hospital staff and visitors as well as patients. The Department of Women's Mental Health Research has incorporated study of the Shedding Skins art and text into several of its student psychology and psychiatry courses. Committed to the Sane Asylum has prompted readers to visit the C A M H exhibit and is available in the C A M H library.

TAKING IT PUBLIC

R O S E M A R Y: Had Susan kept her dream paintings in her home or confined them to discussion with her therapist or with her family and friends, the paintings would have remained an interesting approach to her personal healing, but a private matter. However, Susan was determined to see the paintings installed as a public exhibit. This could have been an exhibit at an art gallery, as befits an artist whose work goes beyond being a personal hobby, and Susan has exhibited at a gallery. But Susan chose to pursue having her paintings installed as exhibits first at Women's College Hospital, then at CAMH. These choices spoke to different purposes and possibilities for her art.

Public events like Susan's that focus on emotional pain and healing provide public windows on these vital, but ordinarily private, experiences, and thus provide opportunities for public discussion. Though the medical model narrative dominates public discussion, other responses to emotional pain thrive, but as narratives that are publically marginal. Healing is often an organizing narrative for individuals and families, but since emotional pain is treated as private, the ways in which individuals or families decide to name and respond to such pain often remain unknown publically.

Public focus on the medical model narrative largely pre-empts discussion of other possibilities. From time to time, public media pieces describe the problems of living with significant emotional pain or otherwise comment on mental illness. Typically such pieces enjoin readers to respond to emotional pain by seeing a doctor, obtaining a diagnosis, and receiving medication. Such media pieces encourage the public to name and respond to emotional pain via the medical model. Occasional media pieces question the medical model. DSM-5 (American Psychiatric Association, 2013) has, for example, been subject to considerable public criticism, including questions about the widespread use of psychoactive medication and the problematic influence of pharmaceutical company marketing programs. However, such critical media pieces generally fail to present any compelling alternative to the medical model for naming and responding to emotional pain. The lack of public visibility for healing, recovery, or other narratives serves to support perception that, flawed though it may be, there are few if any viable alternatives to the illness-focused medical model.

Susan's work demonstrates what can be achieved by making ordinarily private experiences public. Through her art, Susan names her emotional pain in her own terms, for example, "the faceless priest," (see Figure 12.3) rather than in medical model symptoms or diagnoses. She honours the creative, healing capacities within herself by recording and seeking the meaning of her dreams. She finds meaning in experiences that doctors named as illness. She demonstrates the effectiveness of a sustained commitment to well-being. She heals and offers healing stories and images to others. She offers others fresh ways of participating in both her life and their own lives (Barnes 2012). She demonstrates how individuals who have suffered emotional pain contribute to the larger society. In short, her work increases the public visibility of creative, postmodern ways of naming and responding to emotional pain, demonstrates a compelling healing narrative, and thus publically displaces the medical model as the only possible organizing narrative for such pain.

PEOPLE ARE INTERESTED

Susan's Shedding Skins exhibit is one of many public events related to emotional pain. The public is very interested in such events, first because such pain is so pervasive. Who among us has been untouched by it? Emotional pain already makes prominent public appearances under the name "mental illness" and "mental health care," as research studies typically use such constructs when investigating the extent and impact of emotional pain. From such studies, we learn that millions are affected by serious mental illness and that mental health problems are among the leading causes of disability in terms of productive years lost[6] (see also Simmie and Nunes 2001). In other words, emotional pain is widespread and often disabling.

As well, people demonstrate interest in public arts events related to emotional pain by attending or funding such events. In Toronto, for example, theatre performances by transgendered youth have received funding from the Toronto Arts Council, Ontario Arts Council, and Toronto Community Foundation.[7] An expressive arts group for women survivors of violence has, for some years, had annual exhibits at Toronto's Gardiner Museum of Ceramic Art (Thomson 2011), and a three-month retrospective exhibit was held in 2013. Touched by Fire,[8] an online public art exhibit to honour and inspire artists with mood disorder and their families is sponsored by Raymond James, an investment firm, and has had exhibits at the Royal Ontario Museum and other venues. The support provided by government, public institutions, community, and corporate sponsors, and the good audiences attracted to such exhibits, indicate the considerable public interest in events related to emotional pain and healing.

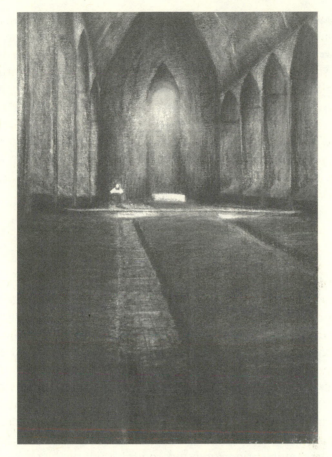

Figure 12.3   Susan Schellenberg, *The Faceless Priest*,
mixed media on paper, 28.75 x 40.75 inches. (Centre for
Addiction and Mental Health, Toronto. Reproduced with
permission)

MEDIA REVIEWS COULD HIGHLIGHT
AND CRITIQUE PUBLIC EVENTS

Media analysis and critical reviews of public arts events relating to
emotional pain could publicize such events, help audiences to
become more knowledgeable, highlight insights, and comment on
how the larger community is invited to perceive and respond to
individuals in emotional pain (Barnes 2012). Some public arts events
seem to publicize illness-focused medical model narratives, for
example, here is how the world looks to people with a certain

diagnosis; here is the mental health victim; here is the rescuer doctor. Reviews could critique the narrow scope or other limitations of
such events. Reviews could explain events that point to healing,
recovery, or other narratives for naming and responding to emotional pain. For example, in *Panopticon*, a 2008 drama produced
by the Central Toronto Youth Services Gender Play program, per-
formers portrayed their own experiences and gave the audience
detailed direction about how to support transgendered youth.
Reviews would likely encourage readers to engage in discussion and
debate about the multiple narratives that can be the basis for
responding to emotional pain.

PUBLIC ARTS EVENTS SUPPORT HEALING
AND REDUCE STIGMA

SUSAN: Writer, storyteller, and friend Helen Porter once said,
"Susan, I am certain if on psychiatric hospital admission someone
had said 'Once upon a time,' followed by a story, you would have
healed much sooner." I painted, wrote, and publically shared my
story long after my psychiatric hospital admission, but those experiences brought the truth of Helen's words to light. Today, I am certain
things would have been different for me if on hospital admission
psychiatrists had said, "Susan, we can easily understand how your
emotional pain may discourage you at this time, but when we see
such pain, we know something in your life has changed. We want to
work with you to bring something positive out of that change. It is
sufferers like you who can help us to help others with similar pain.
We encourage you to believe the mind has a capacity to heal and we
want to share this wellness work with you."

Had psychiatrists used this approach, my 1960s belief that my
badness caused my breakdown would have lessened rather than
flourished into the 1990s. Psychiatric staff reinforced my beliefs of
badness by initially assigning me to a basement ward, then moving
me to wards on progressively higher floors of the building over the
course of my hospital stay. My arrival at a ward on the third floor
indicated my "least bad" state had been achieved and that I was
ready for discharge. Rather than being encouraged to explore recovery tools during my hospital stay, I learned to work a system to gain
my discharge. Later observations of my psychiatric hospital records
confirmed that several of my caregivers had projected badness onto

me, e.g., naming my art as "a bid for approval," and my emotional pain as "a cauldron of snakes."

Had a psychiatrist explained my breakdown as having meaning and purpose, my later passion for healing work convinces me that I would have responded favourably to any "good" theory aimed at replacing my sense of "badness." But no psychiatrist, no fellow patient, no hospital artifact mirrored human goodness back to me in that space. Moreover, anti-psychotic drugs compounded the silence. Until society values and supports more humane approaches to emotional pain than the diagnosis/medication model I experienced, I see my small awareness steps and the publicly shared art and healing stories of others as necessary supports to those whose suffering will mark the minutes as we proceed on that long path to improved societal care.

Where "stigma" is concerned, I believe that publicly shared art and healing stories offer opportunities to highlight the actual contribution that individuals with lived experience can bring to society. Whether the contribution is as large as the founding of Alcoholics Anonymous by Bill Wilson and Dr Bob Smith or as individual as the person who finds the courage to face, resolve, and later to share their story in ways that add to our knowledge of how the mind heals, I feel such contributions must be recognized and honoured. Until this valuing occurs publically as well as privately and individually, current "anti-stigma" campaigns will fail to erase the roots of stigma that lie embedded in the illness-focused medical model narrative.

SUMMARY AND CONCLUSIONS

ROSEMARY: Postmodern and well-being/healing perspectives together suggest effective forms of resistance to the mental illness/medical model narrative. Talking about "emotional pain" helps to keep in mind that "mental illness" or "psychiatric diagnosis" are only a few of the myriad of ways for naming and responding to such pain. An organizing narrative is needed in relation to emotional pain. Narratives that focus on healing, recovery, or other possibilities can provide a reassuring basis to name and respond to emotional pain, but tend to be pre-empted in public discussion by the dominance of the mental illness/medical model. Public arts events such as Susan's Shedding Skins exhibit can effectively direct public attention to healing possibilities for naming and responding to emotional pain; can displace the medical model narrative; and can thus undermine perceptions that medical model care is the only viable response to emotional pain. Public arts events related to emotional pain are particularly important because of the pervasiveness of emotional pain in our society and the considerable public interest in arts events that relate to emotional pain and healing. Media reviews of such events could help to point out underlying narratives and critique the narrow scope of events that encourage involvement only in a mental illness/medical model care. Public arts events can contribute to the healing of both individual artists and others living with emotional pain. Such events also reduce stigma by honouring the ways in which individuals with lived experience of emotional pain contribute to the larger society.

SUSAN: I believe that individuals, along with their communities and environment, benefit when an individual consciously sheds a limiting or harmful behaviour and replaces it with one that brings them closer to compassion for other and self. Unlike the media, which can trigger feelings of being too small and helpless to make a difference in the world, dream and art carry the potential to emphasize our oneness and ability to create change by changing ourselves. In this context, I believe that my artistic work is the radical individual offering to world-making that Gandhi described as, "Be the change you want to see in the world."

My hope for my story and dream art is that they can contribute to contemporary meditations on what it means to heal, and allow others to recall the world and peace-making possibilities of their own dreams.

NOTES

1 A sedative medication.
2 S. Schellenberg and R. Barnes, "Committed to the Sane Asylum: Art as Political Action" (paper presented at PsychoUT: A Conference for Organizing Resistance Against Psychiatry, Ontario Institute for Studies in Education at the University of Toronto, Toronto, 7–8 May 2010), http://individual.utoronto.ca/psychout/abstracts/schellenberg-etal.html. Last accessed 11 May 2012.
3 Schellenberg and Barnes, "Committed to the Sane Asylum: Art as Political Action."

4 In particular, see the strategies for both 2009 and 2012:
   "Toward Recovery & Well-Being: A Framework for a Mental Health
   Strategy for Canada," Mental Health Commission of Canada, 2009.
   http://www.mentalhealthcommission.ca/English/Pages/Reports.aspx.
   Last accessed 30 December 2011.
   "Changing Directions, Changing Lives: The Mental Health Strategy for
   Canada," Mental Health Commission of Canada, 2012. http://strategy.
   mentalhealthcommission.ca/pdf/strategy-text-en.pdf. Last accessed
   15 May 2012.
5 Schellenberg and Barnes, "Committed to the Sane Asylum: Art as Political
   Action."
6 "Out of the Shadows at Last, Transforming Mental Health, Mental Illness,
   and Addiction Services in Canada," Senate Standing Committee on Social
   Affairs, Science, and Technology, 2006. www.parl.gc.ca/39/1/parlbus/com-
   mbus/senate/com-e/soci-e/rep-e/pdf/rep02may06part1-e.pdf. Last accessed
   30 December 2011.
7 N. Brown and L.A. Miller, "Working with Trans Youth: Research and
   Innovative Practice" (paper presented at Children's Mental Health Ontario
   Conference, Toronto, 21 November 2008), www.kidsmentalhealth.ca/doc-
   uments/Res_CTYS_2008.pdf. Last accessed 31 December 2011.
8 "Touched by Fire: A Unique and Exciting Online Gallery of Art by Artists
   with Mood Disorders," Mood Disorders Association of Ontario, 2011.
   http://www.touchedbyfire.ca/. Last accessed 31 December 2011.

13

Feminist Resistance against
the Medicalization of Humanity:
Integrating Knowledge about Psychiatric
Oppression and Marginalized People

SHAINDL DIAMOND

Biological psychiatry is a massive enterprise that is shaped by and interacts with other ruling institutions that are likewise complicit in processes such as colonialism, capitalism, heterosexism, transphobia, ageism, ableism, sexism, adultism, and patriarchy. Within this interconnected web of power, certain marginalized people are particularly vulnerable to psychiatrization.[1] This has been demonstrated in various chapters throughout this book by authors who address various ways that specific marginalized groups are targeted by contemporary psychiatric discourses and practices. Kirby writes about how trans people are forced to interact with the psychiatric system in order to gain access to sex-reassignment surgery, thereby opening them up to the medicalization of their oppression and resistance. LeFrançois addresses how children and youth are disproportionately coerced into relationships with psychiatry against their will, whilst officially appearing on record as 'involuntary' or informal patients. In the next chapter, Mills examines psychiatry as a tool of colonization that enforces dominant notions of normality and "treats" those who do not pass as normal.

As institutional psychiatry grows in power, more and more people are coming into contact with the psychiatric system and are being labeled and subjected to different types of psychiatric intervention. Women and girls coming from diverse social locations are among the most vulnerable in this regard. While there is a long history of women being conceptualized and treated as insane, predating the current period of psychiatric dominance, biological psychiatry is currently the prevailing force that labels and controls the emotional distress and behaviours of women (Burstow 1992; Chesler 1972). There are many disorders listed in the contemporary *Diagnostic and Statistical Manual*, published by the American Psychiatric Association, that are predominantly attributed to women: major depressive disorder; anxiety disorder; somatoform disorder; factitious disorder; dissociative identity disorder, or depersonalization disorder; adjustment disorder; sleep disorder; borderline, histrionic, and dependent disorders; and post-traumatic stress disorder (Becker 2004; Burstow 2005a; Caplan 1995, 2004; Cohen 2004; Fish 2004; Gibson 2004; McSweeney 2004; Rabinor 2004; Ussher 2011). Correspondingly, women are more likely than men to be subject to psychiatric intervention, including institutionalization, accompanied by restraints (Ussher 2011). They are three times more likely to be prescribed electroconvulsive therapy and twice as likely to be given psychopharmaceutical drugs (Burstow 2006a, 2006b; Ussher 2011).

This chapter will look at feminist efforts to depathologize women's responses to trauma and oppression. I argue that these resistance efforts are most effectively understood in the context of a larger struggle against psychiatric oppression – as outlined in various other chapters in this book – and can offer insights that are useful to a larger movement resisting psychiatric oppression and violence. My intention is to demonstrate that feminist contributions are important in any struggle against the medicalization[2] of human experience. At the same time, I set out to address how, at times, feminist efforts have fallen short of questioning more insidious psychiatric theories and practices that pathologize human diversity and responses to trauma. I will explore the importance of working towards a deeper understanding of psychiatric oppression – one that resists the medicalization of human experience in its many diverse forms.

GENDERING MADNESS

Women are not the only gender group subjected to psychiatric labeling and intervention. Emotional, perceptual, and behavioural experiences that are viewed as symptoms of mental illness are experienced by people of many different genders coming from diverse social locations. Nevertheless, madness is a gendered experience, as the ways people feel, perceive, and behave are judged differently depending on gender role expectations (which are in turn shaped by race, class, disability, sexuality, age, and other constructs) associated with the individual's social location (Ussher 2011). Madness is often attributed characteristics that are associated with femininity – the irrational, emotional, weak, and hysterical – and those who are read as mad within dominant culture are associated with these signs of "femininity," whether they are women, men, and/or trans[3] (Chesler 1972). Furthermore, as mentioned earlier, women are more often labeled with psychiatric diagnoses and are more frequently subjected to different types of psychiatric intervention (Burstow 1992, Caplan 2004, Ussher 2011). Some groups of women are at even higher risk of being psychiatrized, including elderly women, girls, racialized women, disabled women, women in prison, trans women, and women living in poverty (Ali 2004; Armstrong 2004; Bullock 2004; Burstow 1992, 2005, 2006; Javed 2004; Jordan et al. 1996; Kilty 2012; Siegel 2004). The increased vulnerability of these women is due to a combination of factors, including the ways in which they disrupt patriarchal hegemony and the contact they may have with institutions (i.e. nursing homes, prisons, schools, medical services, social assistance) that are deeply invested in psychiatry as a means of controlling "deviance."

Feminist critics have frequently emphasized how psychiatric diagnoses ignore structural inequality and oppressive conditions that shape women's experience in favour of individualized conceptualizations of biological deviations that reside in the body (Caplan 1995, 2005; Chesler 1972; Penfold and Walker 1983; Ussher 1991). Many have focused their efforts on deconstructing specific diagnoses, such as major depressive disorder, borderline personality disorder, premenstrual dysphoric disorder, and post-traumatic stress disorder (Burstow 2005a; Caplan 1995, 2005; Shaw and Proctor 2005; Ussher 2011). Rather than understanding women's experiences as a constellation of symptoms that are indicative of mental illness, feminists have reframed these experiences as reasonable responses to material inequities; oppressive gender role expectations that limit women's choices; and pervasive rates of sexual, physical, and emotional abuse (Burstow 1992; Caplan 1995, 2005; Smith and David 1975). They recognize that women respond to oppression, abuse, and violence in a myriad of ways – they cut, they develop problems with eating, they express emotional distress at home or in public, they use substances, and they act angry (Bass and Davis 1988; Blackbridge and Gilhooly 1988; Burstow 1992). These responses are viewed by many feminists as understandable reactions, means of coping, surviving, and resisting oppressive conditions in women's lives (Bass and Davis 1988; Burstow 1992; Smith and David 1975). Challenging the medicalization of women's distress and coping is front and centre in feminist resistance again psychiatric violence and oppression.

Feminists have also emphasized the role of psychiatry as an institution of social control (Burstow 1992; Penfold and Walker 1983; Smith and David 1975). It is viewed as a tool that supports patriarchy by forcing women into the roles of "good wives" and "good mothers" and by silencing their responses to violence and structural inequality (Chesler 1972). One feminist psychiatric survivor who I interviewed, Jackie (cited in Diamond 2012), stated: "Psychiatry is where women end up after they've experienced other forms of violence ... abuse in the family, child abuse, spousal abuse, rape, other assaults ... and when they react ... when they are not functioning, in a way that makes others around them uncomfortable, they are sent to the doctor ... they are drugged, shocked into submission, until they learn to act in a way more comfortable to others." Psychiatric interventions, including diagnosis, psychiatric drugs, electroconvulsive therapy, and institutionalization, are viewed as a means of restraining women who are behaving in ways that disrupt the hegemonic order (Burstow 2006a, 2006b; Chesler 1972). Feminist campaigns have been developed worldwide to resist the targeting of women with psychiatric procedures such as electroconvulsive therapy (Diamond and Weitz 2008; Weitz, Maddock, and Andre 2010). Burstow has named electroconvulsive therapy as a state-sanctioned form of violence against women. Her qualitative research demonstrates how many women experience the threat of electroconvulsive therapy as a coercive tool used to force them into submission (Burstow 2006a, 2006b). Recognizing the lack of support that women often receive when they turn to psychiatry, feminists have developed non-medical services that recognize patriarchal oppression in the lives of women so that they can seek support without being subjected to sexist notions of how to adapt as a "respectable" woman (see also Baker Miller 1986).[4]

The groundwork feminists have laid over the past few decades is
extremely critical in larger discussions about resisting the pervasive
trends of biological psychiatry – trends that affect all of humankind.
Deconstructing the reasons why women experience higher rates
of "symptoms" associated with various diagnoses can help to
shed light on why people of various genders and social locations
might have similar experiences of emotional distress. Understanding
why women experience depression in the context of patriarchal
oppression and violence can provide insight into why many differently situated oppressed people are depressed (Ussher 2011). Such
understandings can illuminate gendered social relations; the ramifi-
cations of inequality and discrimination; and how these cultural,
social, and material realities shape the psychological experience of
humans. Likewise, analyzing how madness is theorized and treated
helps to provide insight into cultural expectations of gender and
gender roles, including what it means to be a respectable "woman"
or "man." Indeed, feminist theorists and activists have offered critical understandings about how psychiatry works to maintain the
hegemonic order, and this work forms an important foundation for
the work differently situated people are doing to depathologize and
protect marginalized people from further psychiatric intrusion
(Becker 2004; Burstow 1992, 2005a; Caplan 1995, 2004; Chesler
1972; Cohen 2004; Fish 2004; Gibson 2004; McSweeney 2004;
Rabinor 2004; Ussher 2011).

DIGGING FOR THE ROOTS
OF PSYCHIATRIC OPPRESSION:
GOING BEYOND SINGLE ISSUE POLITICS

What is concerning is when feminist efforts or the efforts of other
marginalized groups fall short of considering the whole of how psychiatry medicalizes emotional, perceptual, and behavioural experiences. Some feminist theorists offer up in-depth critiques of how
psychiatry enforces gender expectations by punishing women who
deviate from these expectations, but then go on to suggest that
there are some women who are genuinely mentally ill and in need
of psychiatric, psychopharmaceutical, or other types of interventions (Penfold and Walker 1983). Certain diagnoses, such as
schizophrenia, appear to signify true biological fact and are left
untouched by many feminists who are otherwise very progressive

about contextualizing emotional distress and other facets of women's experience.[5] While this critique can be applied to many parts of the feminist movement, there are numerous feminists who challenge this trend. Some feminists are clear that the concept of mental illness itself furthers psychiatric oppression and violence against women and girls, and partake in psychiatric survivor and antipsychiatry initiatives (Burstow 1992, 2005b; Diamond 2012).

The failure to challenge all diagnoses, and the very concept of mental illness itself, reifies the notion that some forms of emotional distress or human experience can be reduced to naturally occurring biological functions in the body. This approach ignores how differences in subjective experiences and bodily functions are socially constructed as "sick," "disabled," "mentally ill," or "in need of correction," and fails to recognize that much of the suffering associated with these very same experiences can and does frequently arise from oppression and trauma. There is of course very real suffering that people experience – emotional distress, anxiety, and pain in the body – but medical discourses designed to support hegemonic power relations largely define how we theorize and interact with these experiences. While most feminists agree that intense sadness, and problems with eating or cutting represent understandable responses to trauma and oppression, many fear alternate experiences of reality or perceptual experiences such as hearing voices and view these experiences as legitimate grounds for physical psychiatric interventions. Treating certain emotional and perceptual experiences as indicative of mental illness separates women from one another and creates further divides among oppressed people of all genders.

The phenomenon of dominant power relations being reproduced in the context of progressive political communities has been studied extensively by Black feminists. Audre Lorde, for example, was among one of the first theorists to describe how these dynamics are reproduced when marginalized people strive to attain the status of the mythical norm, an ideal that is defined as white, able-bodied, hearing, sane, rational, young adult, male, heterosexual, cis-gendered, Christian, middle-class, and thin. Lorde (2007) explains that marginalized people often identify one way in which they are different from the mythical norm and assume this to be the primary cause of oppression, ignoring other misrepresentations of differences, some of which they end up perpetuating themselves. The collective consciousness of political communities is shaped by this mythical norm, and while all people know on some level that they can never attain this norm, they believe that the closer they get to attaining it, the more respectability and power they will gain.

This desire to ascend to the pinnacle to attain the mythical norm creates a hierarchical structure within society that permeates all structures including social movements. This poses major barriers to people coming together, to work in solidarity to challenge systemic oppression at its roots. The question is: why do political communities that are founded on liberation ideologies fall into this trap? Fellows and Razack (1998) assert that it is an act of survival. They argue that people fear their own erasure if they do not continuously prioritize what they see as their primary issue and therefore focus on their own subordination as a self-protective response. In addition, when individuals do not relate to a specific manifestation of oppression, or are even privileged in relation to others as a result of it, they are likely to discount others' claims about injustice, just as dominant groups do when they hear the narratives of marginalized groups (Fellows and Razack 1998).

As Fellows and Razack point out, each individual is privileged by certain dominant representations of the "other," which they use to convince themselves that the "other's narrative" is not as legitimate as their own. To think or feel otherwise, to focus on their own complicity in the oppression of others, is experienced as a threat to their own claims for justice (1998). Where some groups of people are set up to always be constructed as "lesser than" and their oppression is naturalized through the power of the mythical norm, marginalized individuals are pitted against one another in a race for respectability. In the context of feminist efforts to depathologize women, frequently women who have experiences that are not readily understood as resulting from violence are excluded from non-pathologizing frameworks and are left in the hands of psychiatry.

I do not mean to suggest that the process by which certain groups are constructed as inferior is accepted at a conscious level by those who construct some oppressed people as mentally ill and others as sane while oppressed. Rather, this process is often invisible to those who belong to dominant groups, those who are seen as "simply human," and who remain unmarked by identity labels. Fellows and Razack explain: "The marking of subordinate groups and the unmarking of dominant groups leaves the actual processes of domination obscured, thus intact. Subordinate groups simply are the way they are; their condition is naturalized. To be unmarked or unnamed is also simply to embody the norm and not to have actively produced or sustained it. To be the norm, yet to have the norm unnamed, is to be innocent of the domination of others" (1998, 341). In other words, dominant culture conditions individuals to see human differences in simplistic oppositional relationships that are constructed through binaries such as normal/pathological or superior/inferior (Diamond 2006; Lorde 2007; Wilchins 2004). The "normal" subject is always positioned at the centre, while all other subjects who deviate from the mythical norm are relegated to a "lesser than" status. The "normal" is left unquestioned and unscrutinized, while all other subject positions are under constant surveillance and re-evaluation (Wilchins 2004). The processes by which this happens are so ingrained in the organization of the world, so built into language and the foundation of societal institutions, that it creates a situation where individuals within political communities have to work hard to bring them into consciousness and make them visible.

Feminists have made important advances by establishing non-medical counselling services, shelters, and other crisis services for women who have experienced violence (see also Baker Miller 1986).[67] These are invaluable resources for many women who have experienced violence and can save many from entering the psychiatric system by offering them non-medical places to turn to for support. However, even within these services, some feminist practitioners believe that women who they perceive as truly mentally ill are in need of some kind of psychiatric intervention, such as drugs or institutionalization. Therefore, while some women are spared psychiatrization, others who have been previously labeled as mentally ill or who are having alternate experiences of reality are further subjected to psychiatric intervention. For these women, even feminist non-medical services can put them at further jeopardy. Perhaps it feels safer to challenge the medicalization of experiences that are widely recognized as symptomatic of inequality, oppression, and abuse while leaving psychiatric conceptualizations of other experiences left unchallenged. Perhaps this allows for some women to come closer to attaining the status of "normal," thereby gaining more influence within systems of power.

Another complicating factor is that feminist organizations running support services and shelters for women are working with
insufficient or unstable funding and are often unsure of how they
are going to keep their services running. Important feminist organizations have been forced to close their doors in recent times. For
example, the Women's Counselling, Referral, and Education Centre
(WCREC) in Toronto offered services to women, including many
psychiatric survivor women, for many years. This is a feminist organization that actively supported psychiatric survivor and antipsychiatry initiatives. The government cut funding for WCREC, and in
2011, the feminists running this organization were forced to shut
down the critical services they offered. In more conservative political
climates, feminists may be afraid to broaden their analysis in ways
that target psychiatric ideology at its roots. Doing so may mean a
loss of funding for services that are critical in the lives of many
women who have experienced violence.

The ironic aspect of this dynamic is that many women who identify
as psychiatric survivors, including those who are diagnosed with
schizophrenia and those who have alternate experiences of reality,
are abuse survivors (Burstow 1992). Even those who are not abuse
survivors in the traditional sense are subject to insidious forms of
trauma that come from living in a racist, patriarchal, classist, adultist,
ableist, ageist, heterosexist, transphobic, and otherwise oppressive
society (Burstow 1992, 2005a). When these women are psychiatrized,
they are subjected to another form of institutional violence and are
often further traumatized. It is urgent that the feminist movement pay
attention to all women who are survivors of the psychiatric system
and resist letting psychiatric ideology limit the services they offer (or
who they offer services to) or their willingness to pay attention to the
pathologization of a breadth of human experience.

Contextualizing all human experience is a critical step towards
building stronger solidarity networks within and among political
communities that have vested interests in challenging their psychiatric pathologization. Many marginalized people fall into the trap
of distancing themselves from those who they consider to be truly
mentally ill. Several examples appear in this book – in Withers'
chapter, which mentions that some disabled people do not want to
associate with psychiatric survivors, and in Kirby's interview, where
he discusses the efforts of transgender people to separate trans

identities from mental illness, while leaving the concept of mental illness itself unchallenged. Another recurring example in this book is that of the gay rights movement that fought for the removal of the diagnosis of homosexuality from the DSM while failing to consider how many queer people would continue to be psychiatrized for their responses to living in homophobic and heterosexist contexts.[8] It is often the case that individuals associated with marginalized groups do not want to be viewed as "crazy" or "mentally ill" and so distance themselves from people who represent what they accept as true mental illness. They may at times forge strategic alliances with other psychiatrized people, but ultimately, they fear further medicalization of their own oppression.

These examples demonstrate how the gains made by marginalized groups, which aim to achieve the status of the mythical norm for some of the group members, takes place on the backs of those most oppressed in their communities. It is understandable that marginalized groups want to avoid being further pathologized, but in the long run and in the bigger picture, these are not effective strategies. As Fellows and Razack explain, "respectability is a claim for membership of another group; attaining it, even one aspect of it, requires the subordination of Others. Moreover, because subordinate groups that gain a measure of respectability do not by definition possess all the attributes of respectability, they are in an inherently unstable position" (1998, 352). In other words, while oppressed people may feel they are advancing their own claim for justice by differentiating themselves from other oppressed people, by failing to see one's own domination, they are leaving all the systems that privilege them and oppress them intact, and thereby assuring the perpetuation of injustice.

Some marginalized people have come to recognize the interconnectedness of differently situated people's liberation struggles and are digging for the roots of psychiatric oppression. This is evident in certain events targeting psychiatric violence, such as the feminist campaign against electroconvulsive therapy "Stop Shocking Our Mothers and Grandmothers!" Many feminist and disability groups in Canada have supported this campaign and recognize that electroconvulsive therapy needs to be banned so that all people, regardless of how they are situated in relation to psychiatry, are safe from this damaging procedure.

BUILDING AN INTEGRATED FEMINIST RESISTANCE
AGAINST PSYCHIATRY

Audre Lorde argues that it is "the refusal to recognize differences, and to examine the distortions which result from our misnaming them and their effects upon human behaviours and expectation" (2007, 115) that separates us. All people exist within contexts where these distortions shape our living, and it is the systems that create these distortions that are common to all people. Yet in examining the histories of various different groups of marginalized people, interdependence is revealed. It is difficult, for example, for feminists to retain moral credibility while pointing out the psychiatric targeting of women abuse survivors without simultaneously recognizing how racialized survivors of violence are often pathologized as schizophrenic (Metzl 2009; Sharpley and Peters 1999). Similarly, it is problematic for psychiatric survivors to recognize the impact of institutional violence within the psychiatric system without recognizing how racism, sexism, ageism, adultism, heterosexism, transphobia, audism, and ableism put specific groups of marginalized people at greater risk within the system they are critiquing. Additionally, it is very impractical for all of us to ignore the psychiatrization of elderly people, given that most people live to be part of this group. As Hill Collins points out, the same inseparable forces of domination shape the various experiences of marginalized groups, and this recognition "can serve as a foundation for building empathy" among various groups (2000, 247).

Diversity among people resisting psychiatric oppression and violence elucidates the reality that not all people experience psychiatry in the same way. In part, it is this diversity of experiences that people have within the psy-complex (Rose 1999a) that accounts for the different solutions people view as appropriate in their healing, empowerment, and social change work. For example, the racialized woman living in poverty who has been pathologized for how she copes with the insidious trauma of living in a sexist, racist, and classist society may view resistance against racism and classism to be central to her resistance efforts. The woman who is psychiatrized because of how she has responded in the context of an abusive relationship may find the most useful support from feminist antiviolence initiatives. The child living in a group home who is psychiatrized because of her reaction to sexual abuse perpetrated by adults may turn to a children-run organization, such as Youth in Care Canada. The white man who is psychiatrized for hearing voices may find home in a group focused on depathologizing his experiences and offering alternative supports. The trans person who is forced to undergo psychiatric scrutiny in order to access sex-reassignment surgery might be drawn to the development of alternatives in health-care for trans people. Narratives and initiatives that resonate most with an individual's firsthand experience will have the strongest draw, and there is nothing wrong with there being a range of heal-ing, empowerment, and social change initiatives addressing the spe-cific safety needs and desires of particular groups of people.

At the same time, as Black feminist Angela Davis points out, it is important to "be more reflective, more critical" to recognize that "there is often as much heterogeneity" within specific identity groups as within larger communities (cited in James 1998, 299). It is impor-tant to recognize the specificities of experience in order to develop initiatives that meet the needs of different groups of people, as femi-nists working to depathologize and provide services to women sur-vivors of violence have done. It is equally important, though, to allow these differences to lead us to a deeper understanding of connections between us, and to use our understandings of local specificities to theorize universal concerns more thoroughly. By doing so, differently situated people who are resisting psychiatric medicalization can come to recognize how resisting the medicaliza-tion of all identities will benefit us all. This is a necessary part of doing more just and caring work that addresses inequality and the suppression of many forms of oppressed people's resistance. We must stop being complicit in the medicalization and psychiatriza-tion of humankind.

NOTES

1 Psychiatry changes which groups it targets at different moments in history and in different geographic locations. As such, we must continuously re-evaluate which groups in society are at greatest risk of psychiatric intervention.
2 As described by Kilty, medicalization "is a process through which an entity that is not ipso facto a medical problem is responded to as a kind of ill-ness" (2012, 163).

3 I borrow Ambrose Kirby's definition of trans here – to mean "a range of
   identities including but not limited to transsexual, transgender, gender
   queer, gender independent, MTF, FTM, MTM, FTF, transgirl, transboi,
   transman, and transwoman." Like Kirby, I recognize that this terminology
   may not "represent the stories and diversity of all people who identify
   in these ways," but we use it to begin this important conversation.
4 "Women's College Hospital," 2012. http://www.womenscollegehospital.
   ca/programs-and-services/mental-health/. Last accessed 31 October 2012.
5 See the following sources: P. Chesler, "No Safe Place. The Phyllis Chesler
   Organization," (1998). http://www.phyllis-chesler.com/512/no-safe-place.
   Last accessed 31 October 2012. "Brief Psychotherapy Centre for Women,"
   Women's College Hospital, 2012. http://www.womenscollegehospital.ca/
   programs-and-services/mental-health/brief-psychotherapy-centre-for-
   women-%28bpcw%29463/. Last accessed 31 October 2012.
6 "Women's College Hospital" (2012).
7 "Mission Statement."
8 This example dates back as far as the early 1970s when the diagnosis of
   homosexuality was still in the DSM. At this time, gay rights activists were
   fighting for the removal of the diagnosis, arguing that being gay does not
   mean that a person is "mentally ill." While there was some overlap
   between the gay rights movement and the ex-patient movement at that
   time, given the large number of queer people who were labeled and treated
   as mentally ill, the arguments used to depathologize queerness were based
   on, and reinforced, the normal/abnormal dichotomy. In other words, the
   mainstream gay rights movement wanted gay people to be seen as normal,
   respectable members of society, unlike those who were legitimately viewed
   as sick and inferior.
       Finally, in 1973, the diagnosis of homosexuality was removed from the
   DSM due to mounting pressures from the gay and lesbian community and
   changing societal norms. It was replaced with the diagnosis ego-dystonic
   homosexuality, a term used to describe a mental disorder related to the
   distress experienced by many queer people. This diagnosis fails to take
   into account that one can expect to feel distress when associated with an
   identity that is despised in dominant culture. This again left the most marginalized queers behind in the fight for respectability, as many lesbians,
   gay men, and other queer people, who did not fit the mold of the "respectable" gay man or lesbian, were still constructed as sick and abnormal by
   psychiatric discourse and by larger society. While ego-dystonic homosexuality was eventually taken out of the DSM as well, the discourse used to

depathologize gay men and lesbians remains strong and does little to aid the situation of the most marginalized in the queer community. To this day, for example, queer youth who are kicked out of their family homes; those trying to support themselves as sex workers; and those who cope with oppressive conditions by using strategies viewed as deviant, such as drug use, remain marginalized and vulnerable to psychiatrization because of discrimination and their reactions to poverty, racism, homophobia, ageism, ableism, audism, adultism, heterosexism, and sexism.

14

Sly Normality:
Between Quiescence and Revolt

CHINA MILLS

My psychiatrist asked if I heard voices. I answered "No" [a lie]. My psychiatrist was glad to hear that: "Otherwise we would have to hospitalise you in a psychiatric institution," he said.

Ronny, in Romme et al. 2009, 27

When the great lord passes, the wise peasant bows deeply and silently farts.

Ethiopian proverb, cited in Scott 1990, iii

I want to tell you two stories, stories about pretending to agree, pretending to be "sane." The first story is about Marie,[1] she told it to me when I interviewed her about her experiences within the psychiatric system.

MARIE

Marie heard voices for a long time; they helped her and comforted her while her parents sexually abused her. However, sometimes as an adult they caused her distress, usually a sign for her that she was getting stressed or a reminder that she should tell someone about the abuse she experienced as a child and kept secret for a long time afterwards. After a particularly distressing experience she found herself involuntarily hospitalized, face to face with a psychiatrist. She found the courage and told him for the first time she had ever told anyone that she was abused as a child. He told her "she was saying that because she was ill." She made a decision: she knew that this wasn't somewhere she'd get well, so she pretended to comply, pretended to agree, nodded her head to whatever the psychiatrist said, in order to get out as fast as she could.[2]

The second story is about George.

GEORGE

In the 1950s, George, who was labeled as a "chronic schizophrenic," was one of the first people in a psychiatric hospital in the USA to take part in a clinical trial for chlorpromazine (Thorazine); the first neuroleptic to be used in psychiatry, the drug heralded as marking the beginning of pharmaco-psychiatry.

> No one had paid George any attention for years. Now doctors, attendants, and nurses all talked to him and watched eagerly to see what effect the drug would have. His condition improved rapidly. After only two weeks of the drug treatment he was moved to a ward for less disturbed patients where he took part in a number of activities. Soon he was doing so well that he was promoted again. By this time he had lively relationships with the other patients and many members of the hospital staff. He began to spend several hours a day with paints and clays, using them to express the rich fantasy life that had previously interested no one. His doctors marvelled. Attendants praised his skill. George was released from the hospital thirty-eight days after his first dose of Thorazine. While he was signing out he remembered that he had left something behind, went back to his room, and returned with an old sock. The puzzled attendant who asked to see it found thirty-eight Thorazine pills carefully stashed inside the sock. Why, then, had George suddenly come to life? (Dallett 1988, 15)

Pretending to agree, pretending you don't hear voices, pretending to be "normal," pills hidden under tongues, inside cheeks, and inside socks. Psychiatry is haunted by such pretending, by a hidden territory of survival and resistance, like the "infrapolitics" of disguise and deception employed by colonized peoples while they may outwardly appear, in power laden situations, to willingly consent (Scott

1990). While often not read as political, such "keeping secrets and telling lies" (Siebers 2004, 1) marks a "veiled resistance," a troubled "political terrain that lies between quiescence and revolt" (Scott 1990, 197 and 199). This is a space where official constructions of "good adjustment," maintenance, and recovery may work to mask "phantom acceptance" and "phantom normalcy" (Smith 2006, 122).

This chapter is about finding ways to read these stories and strategies of pretending, to see if we can fleetingly glimpse how pretending might disturb our understanding of what it means to be "normal," how pretending might be subversive. This comes out of and connects to a wider project of tracing how the colonial relation is mobilized within psychiatric treatment (Mills 2014). This has the aim of thinking through how the violence of colonialism may enable a rethinking of contemporary forms of psychiatric violence, particularly the construction of certain forms of violence as "natural," "necessary," and "normal" – that is, violence in the name of "treatment" (Mills 2012a). Using post-colonial theory here enables an exploration of how strategies of resistance to colonialism may be read alongside and used to illuminate resistance to psychiatry – resistance that may be secret, sly, covered up. At first I wondered if this pretending is a strategy that has links to "passing," as normal.

PASSING

Passing marks the crossing of lines, of identities, of boundaries. It was first referred to in nineteenth-century US posters offering rewards for runaway slaves who were attempting to pass as white, and thus as "free" (Sollors 1997). Here "passing" meant escape and freedom for enslaved peoples, escape from slavery into a world of white privilege. The literature suggests different typologies of passing, between passing voluntarily with its links to deception and political subversion, and passing almost by accident (Sollers 1997).

There are also many facets of learning to pass; the places out of bounds, "where exposure means expulsion," and the "back places" where concealment is not necessary (Goffman 1963, 102). This partitioning of the world into forbidden, civil, and back places "establishes the going price for revealing or concealing and the significance of being known about or not known about" (ibid., 104). This partitioned world is evident in Scott's account of colonial oppression where the "subordinate moves back and forth ... between two worlds: the world of the master and the offstage world of subordinates" (1990, 191). It can also be read in the experience of occupying other worlds, hearing voices, and dissociating. This concealment is evident in another story:

> A voice hearer is travelling by train from Sheffield to London. He's taken the advice of people in his support group and pinned a small microphone to the lapel of his jacket. This way, he can talk back to his voices and appear to be speaking into a mobile phone. Soon after the train leaves the station, he, like other passengers, begins an animated conversation. Nearing London, the train goes through a series of tunnels. Everyone else loses telephone contact, but he keeps chatting. When the journey ends at St Pancras station, a man comes up to him and says, "I'm sorry to intrude, but I couldn't help noticing that your phone kept working when none of ours did. Could I just ask, what Network are you on?"' (Hornstein 2009, 49)

Seemingly, then, people sometimes pass too well, which hints at why passing held both anxiety and fascination for whites in the nineteenth century Unites States, an anxiety that was muted by the assumption that one could "always tell" (Sollers 1997, 250). While Ronny pretended not to hear voices to avoid hospitalization, for Rosenhan in the 1970s, the opposite was true. Rosenhan[3] and a group of researchers pretended to hear voices in order to be hospitalized, to put psychiatry's assumption that we can "tell the normal from the abnormal" to the test. Psychiatry didn't do so well. Upon telling a psychiatrist that they heard a voice that said "thud," all the participants were admitted to psychiatric hospitals, all then behaved as they usually would, behaved "normally," and many couldn't get out for months. It seemed then that a sane individual could not be "distinguished from the insane context in which he is found."[4] In order to be released the participants had to pretend to agree that they had been ill.

In Rosenhan's study,[5] the researchers passed as voice hearers; they passed, posed, masqueraded as what they were "not really." Thus a passer is usually considered a counterfeit, a pseudo, a phoney, or an impostor (Sollers 1997). But here the "not really" that one passes as suggests that there is a real identity, a "firm and immutable identity" as which one is attempting to pass (Sollers 1997, 250). There's a problem here, then, in relation to passing as sane, for if we assume that the person passing "really" is mentally ill and is secretly passing for what they are not – passing as sane – then this maintains the binary of sanity and insanity.

In the account of passing above, passing is reliant on a prop, it is made possible because of a microphone, a mobile phone "hands free" set. Many of my friends who hear voices have told me stories about the freedom to talk to their voices made possible through mobile phones. Might medication then also be a prop to enable passing? However this is a prop that aims to eradicate the voices, to enable the person to "become" normal, to be assimilated. This seems different to me from passing as white, for while both enable the person whose identity is denigrated to assume an appearance that enables them to access the more privileged position, there is a difference. For while the person who hears voices is able to appear "normal," to blend in using certain props and strategies – these tactics also enable them to hear and speak to the voices that psychiatry and society insist are not really there – to speak to them, slyly. Thus while passing may at times be sly, pretending seems always to be. Is it possible, then, to read the story of pretending another way, a way that disrupts assumptions of a "real" identity, and as a strategy that implies something other than assimilating, adapting? We might read pretending through a post-colonial lens, as a form of mimicry.

"ALMOST THE SAME, BUT NOT QUITE"

Pretending to be normal – mimicking – seems to emerge in the stories of those who have survived the psychiatric system as a tactic, a strategy of deception that enables some freedoms, at a cost. Stories of pretending, of being sly, resonate with Homi Bhabha's framing of mimicry as a key colonial ambivalence, "the desire for a reformed, recognizable Other, as a subject of difference that is almost the same, but not quite" (1994, 85). Constructed around ambivalence, colonial mimicry must, in order to be effective, continually produce its slippage, produce difference. This makes mimicry one of the most "elusive and effective strategies of colonial power" (Bhabha 1994, 85). It is effective because colonial discourse, and arguably psychiatry, frame the colonized (and the mentally ill) as similar to the colonizers, the so-called sane, but not identical. If they were identical then the ideologies that justify colonialism and psychiatry's interventions could not operate, because these "ideologies assume that there is structural non-equivalence, a split between superior and inferior which explains why any one group of people can dominate another at all" (Huddart 2006, 40). However, mimicry, in its very effectiveness, is elusive because of the introduction of difference, of the "almost the same, but not quite." This difference, between normal and abnormal, sane and insane, is "the disturbing distance in-between that constitutes the figure of colonial otherness" (Bhabha 1994, 45). In this between space, between difference and the same, a difference is enabled that cannot be contained, a space is opened up for "something other, a difference that is a little bit uncanny" (ibid., 131). It is here that the agency of the colonized emerges.

MOTTLED AGAINST A MOTTLED BACKGROUND

Lacan says that "Mimicry reveals something in so far as it is distinct from what might be called an itself that is behind" (Lacan 1977, 99). Being distinct from an "itself" behind hints at something more than blending in with the background of normative expectations. For Lacan, nothing of what can be understood as adaptation (behaviour to survive) can be found in mimicry. This is because mimicry operates "strictly in the opposite direction from that which the adaptive result might be presumed to demand," thereby subverting assimilation. Here adaptation to one's background is always bound up with the needs of survival. To mimic one's background "is not a question of harmonizing with the background but, against a mottled background, of becoming mottled." Might we therefore infer that while adaptation solely enables survival, mimicry works in the "opposite direction," as disguise, and as camouflage? Lacan likens this to the kind of camouflage practiced in human warfare – thus suggesting that, more than survival; mimicry is a practice of deception (1977, 99).

One key strategy of mimicry for Bhabha is sly civility, summed up in the Ethiopian proverb "When the great lord passes, the wise peasant bows deeply and silently farts" (1994, 141; cited in Scott 1990, iii). Slyness marks a "turning off" response; it is "the native refusal to satisfy the colonizer's narrative demand," which "represents a frustration of that nineteenth century strategy of surveillance, the *confession*, which seems to dominate the 'calculable' individual by positing the truth that the subject *has* but does not *know*" (Bhabha 1994, 141).

We could read psychiatry then as a form of surveillance, a means to convert the "irrational" into the "calculable" through diagnosis, which posits the psychiatric truth that what some people have, but do not yet know it, is a "mental illness," a "biochemical imbalance." This is a making calculable – or, for Fanon, making "palatable" – of difference (1986, 176).

SLYNESS

Thus we could read pretending to be normal – through hiding pills under tongues and inside socks, through pretending not to hear voices – as a form of sly civility, or sly normality, that disrupts psychiatry's attempts to make people calculable. For Bhabha this slyness is more than a refusal of a narrative demand for the "incalculable," for it produces a problem for colonial codifications, it generates an uncertainty in its refusal to be intelligible, it "changes the narratorial demand itself" (1994, 141).

This refusal to be intelligible through appearing to be intelligible seems different from the "refusal to reproduce hegemonic appearances" discussed by Scott (1990, 203). Pretending to be normal – sly normality – is the opposite of this, as it seems to work not through refusal of, but through the very production of the signs of "normative compliance." It appears to comply, it mimics normality, it fools the eye. It works like the genre of art known as the "trompe l'oeil," which imitates "the depicted object so convincingly that the viewer is momentarily seized by an inability to tell the difference between original and copy, reality and representation" (MacLure et al. 2010, 496). Marie, George, and Rosenhan[6] also "fool the eye" by imitating sanity and insanity so convincingly that for a moment it becomes impossible to tell the difference between them; they mock psychiatry's claims to tell the difference, and raise an anxiety that challenges the integrity of any model that can be mimicked and then discarded so easily.

For Bhabha, this marks an "area between mimicry and mockery," a space that poses an imminent threat to both "normalized" knowledges and disciplinary powers" because it "quite simply mocks its [psychiatry's, colonialism's] power to be a model, that power which supposedly makes it imitable" (1994, 86–8).[7] This has echoes with the strategies of creative self-protection employed by colonized peoples, the "comical imitativeness which indirectly reveals the ridiculousness of the powerful ... an uncanny ability to subvert the valued skills or traits which may ensure one's adaptation to the 'system'" (Nandy 1983, 84). Stories of imitating, pretending, mimicking may enable self-protection because they provide camouflage. Thus mimicry is linked to the visual, to invisibility, faint figures, and partial presence. When Marie pretended to agree with her psychiatrist and when Ronny pretended he didn't hear voices, the penetrative psychiatric gaze was dislocated by this pretence, as a space from which to look back, partially unseen.

For Scott, "the circumspect struggle waged daily by subordinate groups is, like infrared rays, beyond the visible end of the spectrum" (1900, 183). This partialness could itself be a symptom of colonialism and of oppression, of the surveillance of psychiatry. Yet for Fanon, who was pointed at, hailed, through the look of a white child, this surveillance does not make him invisible, it brings him into being as a subject, as a black man:

> "Look, a Negro!" ... I was an object in the midst of other objects ... sealed into that crushing objecthood ... my body suddenly abraded into non-being ... the glances of the other fixed me there ... My body was given back to me sprawled out, distorted ... completely dislocated ... I took myself far off from my own presence, far indeed, and made myself an object. What else could it be for me but an amputation, an excision, a hemorrhage that spattered my whole body with black blood? ... Where am I to be classified? Or, if you prefer, tucked away? (Fanon 1986, 112–13)

"Objectified," "sealed," "abraded," "crushed," "tucked away," this language speaks of the force of colonial subject formation, the spattering of identities that seems to resonate with the formation of psychiatric subjects, the "stickiness,"[8] the for life-ness[9] of psychiatric diagnoses. Peter Bullimore, a psychiatric survivor and voice hearer, was told by his psychiatrist, "you are a chronic Schizophrenic, you will never ever work again, go away and enjoy your life." To him "the words were so damning ... you may as well have just ripped my heart out."[10] An amputation, spattering of black blood, hearts ripped out, this is a language of the psychic violence enacted by colonial and psychiatric systems of forming subjects. Here the violence of colonial and psychiatric subject formation are more deeply entangled than mere analogy, for psychiatry was a key tool of empire, a symbol of "civilization."[11]

Fanon's (1967) encounter alludes to the partitioned partial worlds of the colonized, "a doubling, dissembling image of being in at least two places at once"... a peculiarly colonial condition," like Fanon's black skin, white masks (1986, xvi). The idea of taking yourself from your own presence seems to resonate with stories of how some people use dissociation to escape the trauma of their immediate surroundings. This hints at a way of reading these experiences psychopolitically, which in turn raises the question of how psychic oppression and trauma are interlaced with the socio-economic.

Bhabha's reading of Fanon takes this even further. Fanon's taking himself from his own presence interrupts the interpellating hail,[12] he "defers the object of the look" (Bhabha 1994, 79), the white gaze that spatters his body with black blood. For Bhabha this invisibility, this non-being, in its refusal of presence (its refusal "to be"), interrupts identification and interpellation, and therefore works as a strategy of resistance and subversion, disrupting assumptions of the unitary subject. Such techniques disturb the logic of "specular identification and reveals the performative fictions at the centre of such categories" (Ginsberg 1996, 13).

Such secret arts enable those who enact them to "subvert the perverse satisfaction of the racist, masculinist gaze" that disavows their presence, "by presenting it with an anxious absence, a counter-gaze that turns the discriminatory look ... back on itself" (Bhabha 1994, 67). These disembodied eyes of the subaltern that speak and see from where they are not, disrupt and subvert both the presumed unitary "I" of identity, and the surveillant, disciplinary "eye" of psychiatry. In looking back, unseen, Marie and Ronny could be read post-colonially as subverting the perverse satisfaction of the psychiatric gaze that denies their experiences and delegitimizes their presence. They look back through a counter gaze that turns the discriminatory and delegitimizing look back on psychiatry itself.

For Bhabha there is something particularly feminist in this representation of invisibility as a form of subversion, this veiled resistance in mimicry as a "secret art of revenge" (1994, 80). This is resistance read between the lines. This "veiled resistance" has often not been read as political; however for Scott (1990) it marks a strategy in the "infrapolitics" of subordinated groups, a politics that leaves few traces, that covers its tracks. There is an interlacing and yet also a distinction being made here between invisibility and mimicry, a distinction between invisibility as adaptation (blending in) and invisibility as resistance (being mottled, camouflaged).

The subaltern instance of the slyly normal thus disrupts the boundaries of rationality and normality, and "wreaks its revenge by circulating, *without being seen*" (Bhabha 1994, 79). According to Bhabha these strategies do more than veil resistance – they create a crisis in the representation of personhood that "at the critical moment, initiates the possibility of political subversion" (1994, 79). But how do the partial figures of the colonized and of the slyly normal initiate political subversion? How does a shared critique of power translate into overt political action, and how can it be used to make psychopolitical demands on those in power? We might thus question the scope of resistance made available through postcolonial readings of resistance to psychiatry. Although post-colonial theory may provide useful conceptual tools for exploring and analyzing people's small, often passive acts of resistance, it remains difficult to see how such strategies could have more wide scale sociopolitical significance.

"INFRAPOLITICAL SHADOWS"

Much writing on resistance by oppressed groups assumes that within such groups there is a desire to speak back to the dominant class, an accumulation of pressure from living under unequal conditions. However critics differ in whether this desire is satisfied and thus pacified in the "hidden transcripts" of the oppressed, the "backstage talk," the "offstage discourse of the powerless," and whether these strategies are a substitute for more "real" political resistance (Scott 1990, 184). Some feel these tactics may quell or cool off the desire to resist, and so act as a "relief valve" to preserve the status quo. However, for Scott, this debate presents an abstract situation that assumes one dominant side and one powerless one, when in fact subordination is rooted in material practices connected to appropriation. Thus veiled resistance is enacted through a "host of down-to-earth, low-profile stratagems designed to minimize appropriation," acts such as pilfering, feigned ignorance, shirking, careless labour, secret trade, foot dragging, and poaching – small acts that carried out on a large scale can have widespread economic effects (ibid., 188).

If we then read psychiatrization (the understanding of ever-increasing experiences in psychiatric terms) as a form of colonial appropriation – appropriation of the psychic means of resistance, of personal and political understandings of distress – then we might see sly normality as a strategy to minimize psychiatric appropriation. In Scott's terms, far from "letting off steam" to retain the status quo, such hidden transcripts are "a condition of practical resistance rather than a substitute for it" (ibid., 191). They form the "infrapolitical shadow" that lurks behind every act of open resistance (ibid., 184), a shadow that enables resistance to be sustained in situations where open confrontation is not possible. This speaks to a further need, then, to understand the conditions under which veiled resistance might speak its name and also when open resistance might become veiled (Scott 1990).

Scott explores how the disguised hidden transcript can, in theory, provide the conditions to develop a shared critique of power. Such a critique could lead (and historically has) to the development of networks of solidarity through collectively defined common experiences of, and strategies of resistance to, social inequality and coercive psychiatric treatment. Scott urges us to attend to these offstage political acts of disguise, to enable us to "map a realm of possible dissent" (ibid., 20). A map of the "lies, secrets, silences, and deflections ... routes taken by voices or messages not granted full legitimacy in order not to be altogether lost" (Johnson 1978, 31).

How do we document these experiences and strategies; how do we make such maps without having them rearticulated within the technocratic language of the market (i.e. as manuals where mimicry becomes a coping strategy, available to buy), without them being capitalized upon as new commodities in a global (mental) health marketplace, and without them being rearticulated as new disorders by the pharmaceutical industry within an ever expanding *Diagnostic and Statistical Manual*.

For example, in a recent advertising campaign for Seroquel X R,[13] an anti-psychotic used for "Bipolar Depression," viewers are informed that "Bipolar depression doesn't have to consume you" (presumably if you consume the drug), ending with the caption, "Don't fade, fight."[14] This implies that fading is the opposite of fighting and that in order not to fade (to become visible) one needs to consume medication – Seroquel X R. This sets up a false binary between fading and fighting, as though fading implies that a person is not fighting. This stands in contrast to the potential resistance and subversion implied in being faint, how in fading a person might fight against the normative gaze of psychiatry or pharmacology through their very denial of fully "being"; the disruption of presence. While fading and mimicry might then be strategies for refusing to be interpellated within the neoliberal market economy, they may also be translated by psychiatry as a symptom of an illness to be marketed, a commodity within the very market economy that they (as strategies of resistance) sought to refuse.

"ALMOST ANOTHER SPECIES"

Perhaps, then, we are all pretending to be normal – but seemingly some people occupy the position of having to pretend. They have to pretend to be normal because psychiatric diagnostic systems work to construct certain people as "outside" normality, and outside humanity; a set of people who can be intervened with, rescued, and "treated" by others in their "best interests," with or without their consent (Mills 2012a). Here labels of "irrationality" and experiences constructed in the language of pathology as "symptoms" – such as hearing voices – act as tropes in which humans undergo a suspension of their ontological status as humans (Spandler and Calton 2009). This suspension seems linked to biological explanations of distress, found by Read et al. to be understood by the public as implying that those with a biochemically framed "mental illness" "were fundamentally different or less human," and "almost another species" (2006, 313 and 311). This has strange echoes with colonial constructions of non-Europeans (and particularly women) as either; "ripe for government, passive, child-like … needing leadership and guidance, described always in terms of lack – no initiative, no intellectual powers … or on the other hand … outside society, dangerous, treacherous, emotional, inconstant, wild, threatening, fickle, sexually aberrant, irrational, near animal, lascivious, disruptive, evil, unpredictable" (Carr 1985, 50). Thus colonial constructions of the Orient as backward and wild, populated by irrational, primitive natives in need of civilizing and rescue for "their own good" has its parallels with psychiatry's construction of particular people as irrational, violent, and dangerous.

"EXPECTED TO SEEM NORMAL"

Invisibility, camouflage, and mimicry – the psychological defenses of the colonized (including the psychiatrically colonized) – may undermine psychiatry's attempts at diagnosis and treatment, showing the incomplete character of any civilizing or normalizing project to fully produce a docile body or mind. Yet this resistance seems unable to rearticulate the terms of subject formation insofar as to "thwart the injunction to produce a docile body is not the same as dismantling the injunction or changing the terms of subject constitution" (Butler 1997, 88). It also may do little to get you released from a psychiatric facility. Moreover such secret strategies and tactics can take their toll on people emotionally, meaning that practicing "sly normality" can be hard work: "I find that having psychosis is horrible, but unless I'm acting strangely no one knows and I'm expected to seem normal. I hear very distressing voices all the time and occasionally get weird delusions and see things in a way that other people say are not real. I've been admitted to hospital and sectioned several times because of it."[15] Here the expectation to seem normal may obscure the performance of being slyly normal – how can we tell the difference? Seemingly, in order to be slyly normal, one must always be aware of dominant models of normality and know oneself to be disqualified from them – people must know what "normal" is to be able to "do" it slyly. Thus for Marie to pass as sane, or recovered, to be slyly normal, requires her to know what the norm is, to know that she doesn't fit that norm, and to know that in order to escape the psychiatric gaze she must learn to emulate that norm.

While passing as normal may help secure a place of privilege within the hegemonic, for Titchkosky (2001, online), everything about those whose disabilities or differences are invisible "can be made to signify normalcy" and furthermore these invisible disabilities are "made invisible by the structures and assumptions of normalcy." To make visible these invisible disabilities, to come out as disabled, one must then navigate normative practices of seeing disability, where one may easily be seduced by normal understandings of disability as lack, for example in naming one's difference through a diagnosis (ibid.).

"RESEMBLANCE AND MENACE"

In Loomba's (1998) reading of Fanon, the black person adopts white masks to enable survival and thus "black skin/white masks reflects the miserable schizophrenia of the colonized's identity" (Loomba 1998, 124). Here schizophrenia is deployed as a figure to describe the colonial condition. However it also opens up a reversal, the possibility of reading the colonization at work within the diagnostic category of schizophrenia.

For Fanon it is colonialism itself that is psychopathological, "a disease that distorts human relations and renders everyone within it 'sick'" (Loomba 1998, 122), which hints at the possibilities of a psychopolitical reading of how psychiatry renders increasing numbers of people as sick (Whitaker 2010). Fanon goes on to explore how signs usually interpreted as caused by faulty brain structures within the colonized may mark symbols of resistance. He cites the example of laziness, reading it as marking "the conscious sabotage of the colonial machine" by the colonized (1963, 239). He continues, "The Algerian's criminality, his impulsivity, and the violence of his murders are therefore not the consequences of the organization of his nervous system or of the characterial originality, but the direct product of the colonial situation" (Fanon 1963, 250). Here what psychiatry calls "mental illness" is read as a product of the colonial situation, of inequality, and alienation; furthermore, in its translations of this distress into psychiatric diagnostic categories, psychiatry also alienates, colonizes. This is to read psychiatry critically through a psychopolitical lens, one that for Hook is a move beyond solely blame or emphasis on psychic damage, "towards a strategic consolidation of psychopolitical resources, be those communal (a solidarity of the oppressed) or subjective (a politics of everyday experience)" (2012, 40). In his "in-between" reading, Bhabha is highlighting the disjunction inherent in colonial discourses: that they contain their own undoing, that mimicry is "at once resemblance and menace" (1994, 86). That, "in 'normalizing' the colonial state or subject, the dream of post-Enlightenment civility alienates its own language of liberty and produces another knowledge of its norms" (Bhabha 1994, 86). Marie's pretending, the mimicry of sanity and insanity might then work to produce another knowledge of the normative assumptions of psychiatry, another language "that could help describe the dominant in terms different than its own" (Achuthan 2005, cited in Chakrabarti and Dhar 2009). This has echoes with Gandhi's endorsement of the "non-modern Indian reading of the modern West," which was an attempt to refuse to meet the West's criterion for antagonism (Nandy 1983, 102). In so doing Marie's pretending marks a refusal to meet psychiatry's criterion for what counts as "sane."

This heeds Nandy's (1983, 12) warning that dissent to colonialism was often controlled by the colonizers, who put forward a way of being anti-colonial that was promoted as "proper," "sane," and "rational," making it possible to "to opt for a non-West which itself is a construction of the West." Nandy continues: "Particularly strong is the inner resistance to recognizing the ultimate violence which colonialism does to its victims, namely that it creates a culture in which the ruled are constantly tempted to fight their rulers within the psychological limits set by the latter" (1983, 3). Reading psychiatry as enacting a colonial relation, then, we might trace how it works to set the boundaries of what counts as sane, promoting "sane" and "rational" ways to be anti-psychiatry – an anti-psychiatry that is a construction of psychiatry. Although colonization rarely destroys all creativity and resistance, for Gruzinski "it does succeed more than often in weaving indissoluble ties between indigenous cultures and the imported ones" (cited in Rahnema 1988, 169). Thus while resistance may be sly, so too can be the monopoly of bio-psychiatry as it weaves indissoluble ties between people labeled as mentally ill and medication – ties that are socially and biologically hard to break.

SLY NORMALIZATION

While some people may practice sly normality, techniques of normalization operate slyly and invisibly too. Pharmaceutical companies often do not make adverse and harmful effects of drugs found in clinical trials public; they ghostwrite articles in psychiatric journals to market their products; they pay for psychiatric conferences in exotic locations (Healy 2006, Moncrieff 2003). I have heard many stories about the effects of taking psychiatric medications; of drooling, of forgetting things, of not being able to recognize the faces of friends. What happens, then, when medication enters the performance of sly normality? How "sly" can you be when, as Pete

told me he had felt while in a psychiatric hospital, you are so heavily medicated that you're like a "zombie," when you can't think
anymore and find it exhausting to speak. And what about if small
doses of medication enable people to be sly, help them to pretend in
order to escape the psychiatric gaze and then stop taking the medication given to them by psychiatrists? Or does medication work to
make people visible, to prevent slyness? Is it possible to be sly in
psycho-pharmaceutical spaces?

How can we know if pretending to be normal is sly, and whether
sly normality resists psychiatry within its own limits, remaining an
"homage to the victors" (Nandy 1983, 12)? Sly normality as a hidden transcript, an infra-political strategy of resistance (Scott 1990),
thus leads us into a new terrain; one that is partial, secret, almost
invisible, but not quite. But with what tools can we recognize and
"see" sly normality? If mimicry and slyness provide camouflage –
invisibility – born of an awareness of unequal power relations, what
are the ethics of "seeing" it? If we "see" it, does this not diminish its
subversive potential, the partial visibility central to it as a strategy
of resistance? Or is it in the breaking of the illusion that subversion
may lie? How can we encounter sly normality without capitalizing
on it, without assimilating it? And when we do encounter it, how do
we know if it is not recuperating the norm: how do we know if it's
subversive? We will never know the number of pills hidden under
tongues and inside socks. This is sly normality as ambivalence, as
seduction, as symptom of oppression, and as subversion.

NOTES

1 All names have been changed throughout (unless specified) to ensure
   anonymity.
2 Story told to me during a piece of research titled "Young People's Stories
   about Hearing Voices" funded by Research Institute of Health and Social
   Change (RIHSC), at Manchester Metropolitan University (MMU),
   December 2007–March 2008.
3 D. Rosenhan, "On Being Sane in Insane Places," (1973). http://psychrights.
   org/articles/rosenham.htm. Last accessed 28 June 2012.
4 "On Being Sane in Insane Places."
5 Ibid.
6 Ibid.

7 This space between mimicry and mockery also seems to be at work in spoof/fake adverts for psycho-pharmaceuticals; see C. Mills (2012b).

8 "On Being Sane in Insane Places."

9 I. Tucker, "'This is for Life': A Discursive Analysis of the Dilemmas of Constructing Diagnostic Identities," *Forum: Qualitative Social Research (FQS)* 10, no. 3 (2009): Article 24. http://www.qualitative-research.net/index.php/fqs/article/view/1376/2872. Last accessed 12 September 2010.

10 From an interview with Peter Bullimore as part of a research project, funded by the Research Institute of Health and Social Change (RIHSC), at Manchester Metropolitan University (MMU), December 2007–March 2008.

11 For a more detailed exploration of the intertwining of psychiatric, and colonial, systems of subject formation, please see Mills, 2014.

12 This draws upon Althusser's (1971) formulation of interpellation, which occurs when a subject turns in answer to a shout in the street, similar to the banal, everyday act of a police officer hailing a person – "Hey, you there!" And by turning, the subject becomes the "you there," meaning they come into being through being hailed by an ideology.

13 "Seroquel XR Advertisement," Seroquel XR, 2010. http://www.youtube.com/watch?v=ictonupsrbo. Last accessed 27 September 2011.

14 Ibid.

15 P. Byrne, "Managing the Acute Psychotic Episode," *Clinical Review, British Medical Journal* 334 (2007): 690. http://www.bmj.com/cgi/content/extract/334/7595/686. Last accessed 22 May 2010.

References

Abbey Strowger, M. 2009. "Time After Time: The 'Doings' of Anxiety's Appearance in the World." Paper presented at the Society for Disability Studies Annual Conference, Tucson, Arizona, 17–20 June 2009.

Abbott, D., and J. Howarth. 2005. *Secret Loves, Hidden Lives? Exploring Issues for People with Learning Difficulties Who Are Gay, Lesbian or Bisexual*. Bristol: Policy Press.

Abdallah, C., C.I. Cohen, M. Sanchez-Almira, P. Reyes, and P. Ramirez. 2009. "Community Integration and Associated Factors among Older Adults with Schizophrenia." *Psychiatric Services* 60: 1642–8.

Ahmed, S. 1998. "Ethics." In *Differences That Matter: Feminist Theory and Postmodernism*, 45–67. Cambridge: Cambridge University Press.

– 2004. "The Contingency of Pain." In *The Cultural Politics of Emotion*, 20–41. New York: Routledge.

– 2006. "The Non-performativity of Anti-racism." *Borderlands E-journal* 5, no. 3. http://www.borderlands.net.au/vol5no3_2006/ahmed_nonperform.htm. Last accessed 10 October 2012.

Alexander, M. 2012. *The New Jim Crow: Mass Incarceration in the Age of Colorblindness*. New York: The New Press.

Ali, A. 2004. "The Intersection of Racism and Sexism in Psychiatric Diagnosis." In *Bias in Psychiatric Diagnosis*, edited by P. Caplan and L. Cosgrove, 71–6. New York: Jason Aronson.

al Nakba, T. 2008. "The Forgotten Spirits of Rabinal." http://upside down-world.org/main/guatemala-archives-33/1442-guatemala-the-forgotten-spirits-of-rabinal. Last accessed 10 October 2012.

Alwood, E. 1996. *Straight News: Gays, Lesbians, and the News Media*. New York: Columbia University Press.

Andreasen, N.C. 1985. *The Broken Brain: The Biological Revolution in Psychiatry*. New York: Harper & Row.

American Psychiatric Association (APA). 1973. *Homosexuality and sexual orientation disturbance: Proposed change in DSM-II, 6th printing, page 44 Position Statement (Retired)*. (Document Reference No. 730008). Arlington: American Psychiatric Association.

– 1980. *Diagnostic and Statistical Manual of Mental Disorders (DSM)*, third edition. Washington: American Psychiatric Association.

– 2000. *Diagnostic and Statistical Manual of Mental Disorders*, fourth edition. Washington: American Psychiatric Association.

– 2013. *Diagnostic and Statistical Manual of Mental Disorders*, fifth edition. Arlington: American Psychiatric Association.

Arendt, H. 1964. *Eichmann in Jerusalem*. New York: Viking Press.

– 1998. *The Human Condition*. Chicago: The University of Chicago Press.

Armstrong, L. 2004. "The Psychiatric Policing of Children." In *Bias in Psychiatric Diagnosis*, edited by P. Caplan and L. Cosgrove, 99–108. New York: Jason Aronson.

Bach, S. 2010. "Public Sector Industrial Relations: The Challenge of Modernization." In *Industrial Relations – Theory and Practice*, edited by T. Colling and M. Terry, 151–77. Chichester: John Wiley.

Badiou, A. 2001. *Ethics: An Essay on the Understanding of Evil*. London: Verso.

Bahm, A., and C. Forchuk. 2008. "Interlocking Oppressions: The Effect of a Comorbid Disability on Perceived Stigma and Discrimination among Mental Health Consumers in Canada." *Health and Social Care in the Community* 17, no. 1: 63–70.

Baker Miller, J. 1986. *Toward a New Psychology of Women*, 2nd edition. Boston: Beacon.

Bangay, F. 2000. "An Uphill Struggle, But It's Been Worth It." In *Mad Pride: A Celebration of Mad Culture*, edited by T. Curtis, R. Dellar, E. Leslie, and B. Watson, 101–4. London: Chipmunkapublishing.

Barnes, C., G. Mercer, and T. Shakespeare. 1999. *Exploring Disability: A Sociological Introduction*. Cambridge: Polity Press.

Barnes, M. 2008. "Passionate Participation: Emotional Experiences and Expressions in Deliberative Forums." *Critical Social Policy* 29: 374–97.

Barnes, M., and P. Cotterell. 2012. "Introduction: From Margin to Mainstream." In *Critical Perspectives on User Involvement*, edited by M. Barnes and P. Cotterell, xv–xxvi. Bristol: Policy Press.

Barnes, M., J. Newman, and H. Sullivan. 2007. *Power, Participation, and Political Renewal: Case Studies in Public Participation*. Bristol: Policy Press.

Barnes, R.A. 2012. "Take it Public: Exhibiting, Performing, and Critiquing Expressive Arts." *Canadian Art Therapy Journal* 25: 1–6.

Barnes, R.A., and S. Schellenberg. 2004. "The Pleasures of Healing, the Possibilities for Mental Health Care." *Canadian Women's Studies/les cahiers de la femme* 24: 194–9.

Baron, C. 1987. *Asylum to Anarchy*. London: Free Association Books.

Bass, E., and L. Davis. 1988. *The Courage to Heal: A Guide for Women Survivors of Child Sexual Abuse*. New York: Harper & Row.

Beal, G., G. Veldhorst, J. McGrath, S. Guruge, P. Grewal, R. DuNunzio, and J. Trimnell. 2005. "Constituting Community: Creating a Place for Oneself." *Psychiatry* 68, no. 3: 199–211.

Becker, D. 2004. "Post-traumatic Stress Disorder." In *Bias in Psychiatric Diagnosis*, edited by P. Caplan and L. Cosgrove, 207–12. New York: Jason Aronson.

Bendell, K., J. Sylvestre, A. Wright, E. Kristjansson, and J. Cousins. 2010. *Using Photovoice to Understand Experiences of Supportive Housing in Ottawa*. Ottawa: Canada Mortgage and Housing Corporation.

Bentall, R.P., ed. 1990. *Reconstructing Schizophrenia*. New York: Routledge.

Beresford, P. 2002. "User Involvement in Research and Evaluation: Liberation or Regulation?" *Social Policy & Society* 1, no. 2: 95–105.

Beresford, P. 2005a. "'Service User': Regressive or Liberatory Terminology? Current Issues." *Disability & Society* 20, no. 4: 469–77.

– 2005b. "Social Approaches to Madness and Distress: User Perspectives and User Knowledges." In *Social Perspectives in Mental Health: Developing Social Models to Understand and Work with Mental Distress*, edited by J. Tew, 32–52. London: Jessica Kingsley Publishers.

– 2010. "Public Partnerships, Governance, and User Involvement: A Service User Perspective." *International Journal of Consumer Studies* 34, no. 5: 495–502.

Beresford, P., and P. Campbell. 2004. "Participation and Protest: Mental Health Service Users/Survivors." In *Democracy and Participation: Popular Protest and New Social Movements*, edited by M.J. Todd and G. Taylor, 326–42. London: Merlin Press.

Beresford, P., G. Gifford, and C. Harrison. 1996. "What has Disability Got to Do with Psychiatric Survivors? In *Speaking Our Minds: An Anthology of Personal Experience of Mental Distress and Its Consequences*, edited by J. Read and J. Reynolds, 209–14. Basingstoke: Macmillan/Palgrave.

Beresford, P., M. Nettle, and R. Perring. 2009. *Towards A Social Model Of Madness and Distress?: Exploring What Service Users Say*, 22 November. York: Joseph Rowntree Foundation.

Bhabha, H.K. 2005 [1994]. *The Location of Culture*. London and New York: Routledge.

– 1986. Forward to *Black Skin, White Masks*, Frantz Fanon, vii–xxvi. London: Pluto Press.

Blackbridge, P., and S. Gillhooly. 1985. *Still Sane*. Vancouver: Press Gang.

– 1988. "Still Sane." In *Shrink Resistant: The Struggle Against Psychiatry in Canada*, edited by B. Burstow and D. Weitz, 44–51. Vancouver: New Star Books.

Bourdieu, P. 1990. *The Logic of Practice*. Stanford: Stanford University Press.

Bracken, P., and P. Thomas. 2005. *Postpsychiatry: Critical Perspectives on Recovery*. Oxford: Oxford University Press.

Branfield, F. 2009. *Developing User Involvement in Social Work Education*. SCIE Report 29. London: Social Care Institute for Excellence.

Branfield, F., P. Beresford, and E. Levin. 2007. *Common Aims: A Strategy to Support Service User Involvement in Social Work Education*. London: Social Care Institute for Excellence.

Breeding, J., and E. Scogin. 2012. "One Woman's Near Destruction and Reemergence from Psychiatric Assault: The Inspiring Story of Evelyn Scogin." *Journal of Humanistic Psychology* 52, no. 1: 53–72.

Breggin, P.R. 1979. *Electroshock: Its Brain-Disabling Effects*. New York: Springer.

– 1991. *Toxic Psychiatry*. New York: St Martin's Press.

– 1997. *Brain-disabling Treatments in Psychiatry: Drugs, Electroshock, and the Role of the FDA*. New York: Springer.

– 2008. *Brain-disabling Treatments in Psychiatry: Drugs, Electroshock, and the Psychopharmaceutical Complex*, 2nd edition. New York: Springer.

Brennan, M.V. Forrest, and J. Taylor. 2012. "Involving People with Learning Difficulties and Self Advocacy." In *Social Care Service Users and User Involvement*, edited by P. Beresford and S. Carr, Research Highlights 55, 249–64. London: Jessica Kingsley Publishers.

Bronski, M. 1984. *Culture Clash: The Making of Gay Sensibility*. Boston: South End Press.

Brown, H., and H. Smith. 1992. "Assertion, Not Assimilation: A Feminist Perspective on the Normalisation Principle." In *Normalisation: A*

Reader for the Nineties, edited by H. Brown and H. Smith, 149–69.
New York: Routledge.

Brown, W. 1995. *States of Injury: Power and Freedom in Late Modernity*.
Princeton: Princeton University Press.

– 2000. "Suffering Rights as Paradoxes." *Constellations* 7, no. 2: 230–41.

Bruner, A. 1963. "C A S: 'Backbone' of Ontario Child Welfare." *Toronto
Star*, 15 July.

Bullock, H.E. 2004. "Diagnosis of Low-income Women." In *Bias in
Psychiatric Diagnosis*, edited by P. Caplan and L. Cosgrove, 115–20.
New York: Jason Aronson.

Burstow, B. 1990. A "History of Psychiatric Homophobia." *Phoenix
Rising* (July): S38–9.

– 1992. *Radical Feminist Therapy: Working in the Context of Violence*.
Newbury Park: Sage Publications.

– 2003. "Toward a Radical Understanding of Trauma and Trauma Work."
Violence against Women 10, no. 11: 293–317.

– 2005a. "A Critique of Posttraumatic Stress Disorder and the D S M."
Journal of Humanistic Psychology 45, no. 4: 429–45.

– 2005b. "Feminist Antipsychiatry Praxis: Women and the movement(s)."
In *Women, Madness, and the Law: A Feminist Reader*, edited by W.
Chan, D. Chunn, and R. Menzies, 245–58. London: Glasshouse.

– 2006a. "Electroshock as a Form of Violence against Women." *Violence
against Women* 12, no. 4: 372–92.

– 2006b. "Understanding and Ending E C T: A Feminist Perspective."
Canadian Woman Studies 25, nos. 1 and 2: 115–22.

Burstow, B., L. Cohan, B. Diamond, et al. 2005. *Report of the Psychiatric
Drug Panel*. Toronto: Inquiry into Psychiatry.

Butler, J. 2004. *Precarious Life*. New York: Verso.

Cairney, R. 1996. "'Democracy Was Never Intended for Degenerates':
Alberta's Flirtation with Eugenics Comes Back to Haunt It." *Canadian
Medical Association Journal* 155, no. 6: 789–92.

Campbell, J. and M. Oliver. 1996. *Disability Politics: Understanding Our
Past, Changing Our Future*. London: Routledge.

Campbell, L.A., M. Cox, S. Kisely, D. Lawrence, S. Maate, and M. Smith.
2007. "Inequitable Access for Mentally Ill Patients to Some Medically
Necessary Procedures." *Canadian Medical Association Journal* 176,
no. 6: 779–88.

Campbell, P. 2009. "The Service User/Survivor Movement." In *Mental
Health Still Matters*, edited by J. Reynolds, R. Muston, T. Heller,

J. Leach, M. McCormick, J. Wallcraft, and M. Walsh, 218–25.
Basingstoke: Palgrave/Open University Press.

Canguilhem, G. 2011 [1958]. "What is Psychology?" In *Critical Psychology: Critical Concepts in Psychology*, edited by I. Parker, vol. 1, 416–28. London and New York: Routledge.

Caplan, E.J. 2004. "Psychiatric Diagnosis in the Legal System." In *Bias in Psychiatric Diagnosis*, edited by P. Caplan and L. Cosgrove, 49–34. New York: Jason Aronson.

Caplan, P. 1995. *They Say You're Crazy: How the World's Most Powerful Psychiatrist Decides Who's Normal*. Reading: Perseus Books.

– 2005. *The Myth of Women's Masochism*. Scarborough: New American Library of Canada.

Caplan, P. and L. Cosgrove, eds. 2004. *Bias in Psychiatric Diagnosis*. New York: Jason Aronson.

Capponi, P. 1992. *Upstairs in the Crazy House: The Life of a Psychiatric Survivor*. Toronto: Viking.

Carr, H. 1985. "Woman/Indian, the 'American' and His Others." In *Europe and its Others*, vol. 2, edited by F. Barker, P. Hulme, M. Iversen, and D. Loxley, 46–60. Colchester: University of Essex Press.

Center for the Human Rights of Users and Survivors of Psychiatry (CHRUSP). 2009. http://www.chrusp.org/home. Last accessed 22 October 2012.

Chakrabarti, A. and A. Dhar. 2010. *Dislocation and Resettlement in Development*. London and New York: Routledge.

Chamberlin, J. 1990. "The Ex-patients Movement: Where We've Been and Where." *The Journal of Mind and Behaviour* 11, nos. 3 and 4: 323–36.

Chan, W., D. Chunn, and R. Menzies, eds. 2005. *Women, Madness, and the Law: A Feminist Reader*. London: The Glass House Press.

Chaplin, J., and C. Haggart. 1983. *The Mass Psychology of Thatcherism*. London: West London Socialist Society.

Chapman, C. 2007. "Dilemmas about 'Taking Responsibility' and Cultural Accountability in Working with Men Who Have Abused their Female Partners." *The International Journal of Narrative Therapy and Community Work* 4: 58–62.

– 2009. "Self-reflexive Critique and Fostering Communities of Support in Education for Social Change." Paper presented at Education Spaces/Places: Exploring the Boundaries of Adult Education: 28th Annual Conference Proceedings of the Canadian Association for the Study of Adult, Ottawa, 326–8. http://www.casae-aceea.ca/sites/casae/archives/

cnf2009/OnlineProceedings-2009/CASAE2009%20Proceedings%20
TOC.html#Roundtables. Last accessed 10 October 2012.

— 2010a. "Crippling Narratives and Disabling Shame: Disability as a
Metaphor, Affective Dividing Practices, and an Ethics that Might Make
a Difference." Paper presented at The Space between: Disability in and
Out of the Counselling Room Conference, Toronto, 8 October 2010.

— 2010b. "Using Our Everyday Ethical Transgressions as Starting Points
for Social Justice Education." *Canadian Association for the Study of
Adult Education*, Montreal. http://www.casae-aceea.ca/sites/casae/
archives/cnf2010/OnlineProceedings-2010/CASAEcnf2010-Proceedings.
html. Last accessed 10 October 2012.

— 2011. "Resonance, Intersectionality, and Reflexivity in Critical Pedagogy
(and Qualitative Research)." *Social Work Education* 30, no. 7: 723–44.

— 2012. "Colonialism, Disability, and Possible Lives: The Residential
Treatment of Children Whose Parents Survived Indian Residential
Schools." *The Journal of Progressive Human Services* 24, no. 2: 127–58.

Chesler, P. 1972. *Women and Madness*. New York: Avon.

— 2005. *Women and Madness*, revised edition. Houndmills: Palgrave
Macmillan.

Chomsky, N. 2012. *Occupy*. New York: Zuccotti Park Press.

Chrisjohn, R., S. Young, and M. Maraun. 2006. *The Circle Game: Shadows
and Substance in the Indian Residential School Experience in Canada*.
Penticton: Theytus Books.

Church, K. 1995. *Forbidden Narratives: Critical Autobiography as Social
Science*. London: Routledge.

— 2013. "Making Madness Matter in Academic Practice." In *Mad Matters:
A Critical Reader in Canadian Mad Studies*, edited by B.A. LeFrançois,
R. Menzies, and G. Reaume, chapter 13. Toronto: Canadian Scholars'
Press.

Clarke, J. 2007. "Citizen-consumers and Public Service Reform: At the
Limits of Neoliberalism?" *Policy Futures in Education* 5: 239–248.

Cohen, E. 2004. "The Fine Line between Clinical and Subclinical
Anorexia." In *Bias in Psychiatric Diagnosis*, edited by P. Caplan and
L. Cosgrove, 193–200. New York: Jason Aronson.

Colbert, T. 2001. *Rape of the Soul*. Tustin: Kevco.

Coleman, E. 2008. "The Politics of Rationality: Psychiatric Survivors'
Challenge to Psychiatry." In *Tactical Biopolitics: Art, Activism, and
Technoscience*, edited by B. Da Costa and K. Philip, 341–63. Cambridge:
The MIT Press.

Collier, R. 2009. "Fatherhood, Law, and Fathers' Rights: Rethinking the Relationship between Gender and Welfare." In *Rights, Gender, and Family Law*, edited by J. Herring, S. Choudry, and J. Wallbank, 119–43. London: Routledge Cavendish.

Cook, J., and J.A. Jonikas. 2002. "Self-determination among Mental Heath Consumers/Survivors: Using Lessons from the Past to Guide the Future." *Journal of Disability Policy Studies* 13, no. 2: 87–95.

Cooke, B., and U. Kothari. 2002. *Participation: The New Tyranny?* London: Zed Books.

Conrad, P. 2007. *The Medicalization of Society: On the Transformation of Human Conditions into Treatable Disorders.* Baltimore: Johns Hopkins University Press.

Corrigan, P., and A. Watson. 2002. "The Paradox of Self-Stigma and Mental Illness." *Clinical Psychology: Science and Practice* 9, no. 1: 35–53.

Cran, B., and G. Jerome. 2008. *Hope in Shadows: Stories and Photographs of Vancouver's Downtown East Side.* Vancouver: Pivot Legal Society.

Cresswell, M. 2009. "Deeply Engaged Relationships? Community Trade Unionism and Mental Health Movements in the UK." Lead Address to Fringe Meeting – Unison in the Community: Mutuality and Solidarity. Unison Health Conference, Harrogate, 20–22 April.

Cresswell, M., and H. Spandler. 2009. "Psychopolitics: Peter Sedgwick's Legacy for the Politics of Mental Health." *Social Theory & Health* 7, no. 2: 129–47.

Crossley, N. 1999. "Fish, Field, Habitus, and Madness: The First Wave Mental Health Users Movement." *British Journal of Sociology* 50: 647–70.

– 2004. "On Systematically Distorted Communication: Bourdieu and the Socio-analysis of Publics." *The Sociological Review. Special Issue – After Habermas: New Perspectives on the Public Sphere* 52, special issue 1: 88–112.

Crouch, C. 2011. *The Strange Non-death of Neoliberalism.* Cambridge: Polity Press.

Dallett, J. 1988. *When the Spirits Come Back.* Toronto: Inner City Books.

Daley A., L. Costa, and L. Ross. 2012. "(W)righting Women: Constructions of Gender, Sexuality, and Race in the Psychiatric Chart." *Culture, Health, and Sexuality: An International Journal for Research, Intervention, and Care* 14, no. 8: 955–69.

Daly, K., and J. Stubbs. 2005. "Feminist Engagement with Restorative Justice." *Theoretical Criminology* 10, no.1: 9–28.

Davidson, L., C. Harding, and L. Spaniol. 2005a. *Recovery from Severe Mental Illnesses: Research Evidence and Implications for Practice, Vol. 1.* Boston: Center for Psychiatric Rehabilitation, Boston University.

– 2005b. *Recovery from Severe Mental Illnesses: Research Evidence and Implications for Practice, Vol. 2.* Boston: Center for Psychiatric Rehabilitation, Boston University.

Davidson, L., M.J. O'Connell, J. Tondora, M. Lawless, A. C. Evans. 2005. "Recovery in Serious Mental Illness: A New Wine or Just a New Bottle?" *Professional Psychology: Research and Practice* 36: 480–7.

Davis, A.Y. 1988. "Coalition Building Among People of Color: A Discussion with Angela Y. Davis and Elizabeth Martinez." In *The Angela Y. Davis Reader*, edited by J. James, 297–306. Malden: Blackwell.

– 2007. "How Does Change Happen?" http://www.youtube.com/watch?v=Pc6RHtEbiOA&feature=related. Last accessed 10 October 2012.

Dean, M. 1999. *Governmentality: Power and Rule in Modern Society.* London: Sage.

Dear M., and J. Wolch. 1987. *Landscapes of Despair: From Deinstitutionalization to Homelessness.* Oxford: Polity Press.

Derrida, J. 1995. *The Gift of Death.* Chicago: University of Chicago Press.

Deverteuil, G. 2011. "Evidence of Gentrification-induced Displacement among Social Services in London and Los Angeles." *Urban Studies* 48, no. 8: 155–71.

De Vos, J. 2012. *Psychologisation in Times of Globalisation.* London and New York: Routledge.

Dhand, R. 2011. "Access to Justice for Ethno-Racial Consumer/ Survivors in Ontario." *Windsor Year Book of Access to Justice* 29: 127–62.

Diamond, S. 2006. "Queer Theory, Gender Theory." *Lesbian & Gay Psychology Review* 7, no. 2: 239–45.

– 2012. "Against the Medicalization of Humanity: A Critical Ethnography of a Community Trying to Build a World Free of Sanism and Psychiatric Oppression." PhD Thesis, University of Toronto.

– 2013. "What Makes Us a Community? Reflections on Building Solidarity in Anti-Sanist Praxis." *Mad Matters: A Critical Reader in Canadian Mad Studies*, edited by B.A. LeFrançois, R. Menzies, and G. Reaume, chapter 4. Toronto: Canadian Scholars' Press.

Diamond, S., and D. Weitz. 2008. "End Electroshock Now: Contemporary Resistance Against Electroshock in Canada." Paper presented at Madness, Citizenship, and Social Justice: A Human Rights Conference, Vancouver, 12–15 June 2008.

Dick, L. 1995. "'Pibloktoq' (Arctic Hysteria): A Construction of European-Inuit Relations?" *Arctic Anthropology* 32, no. 2:1–42.

Dragiewicz, M. 2008. "Patriarchy Reasserted: Fathers' Rights and Anti-VAWA Activism." *Feminist Criminology* 3:121–44.

Drinkwater, C. 2005. "Supported Living and the Production of Individuals." In *Foucault and the Government of Disability*, edited by S. Tremain, 229–44. Ann Arbor: University of Michigan Press.

Du Bois, W.E.B. 2005 [1903]. *The [Illustrated] Souls of Black Folk*. Boulder: Paradigm Publishers.

Dyjur, L., J. Rankin, and A. Lane. 2011. "Maths for Medications: An Analytical Exemplar of the Social Organization of Nurses' Knowledge." *Nursing Philosophy* 12, no. 3: 200–13.

– 2010. *Electroshock: Position of the PsychoUT Conference: A Proposal to Be Considered at the Plenary*. Toronto: PsychoUT Conference.

Esterberg, K.G. 1990. "From Illness to Action: Conceptions of Homosexuality in the Ladder, 1956–1965." *Journal of Sex Research* 27, no. 1: 65–80.

Esther, L. 2003. "Mad Pride and Prejudice." In *Mad Pride: A Celebration of Mad Culture*, edited R. Deller, T. Curtis, and Leslie Esther. Toronto: Chipmunkapublishing.

Everett, B. 2000. *A Fragile Revolution: Consumers and Psychiatric Survivors Confront the Power of the Mental Health System*. Waterloo: Wilfred Laurier University Press.

Fellows, M.L., and S. Razack. 1998. "The Race to Innocence: Confronting Hierarchical Relations among Women." *Journal of Gender, Race, and Justice* 1: 335–52.

Fabris, E. 2006. "Identity, Inmates, Insight, Capacity, Consent: Chemical Incarceration in Psychiatric Survivor Experiences of Community Treatment Orders." MA Thesis, University of Toronto.

Fanon, F. 1968. *Black Skin, White Masks*. New York: Grove Press.

Fenby, B.L. 1991. "The Community Residence as a Family: In the Name of the Father." *Journal of Independent Social Work* 5, no. 3/4: 121–34.

Filc, D. 2004. "The Medical Text: Between Biomedicine and Hegemony." *Social Science & Medicine* 59, no. 6: 1275–85.

Filion, P. 2000. "Balancing Concentration and Dispersion? Public Policy and Urban Structure in Toronto." *Environment and Planning C* 18: 163–89.

Finkelstein, V. 2002 [1991]. "'We' Are Not Disabled, 'You' Are." In *Constructing Deafness*, edited by S. Gregory and G.M. Hartley, 265–71. London: Continuum.

Finkler, L. 2006. "Re-Placing (In) Justice: Disability-Related Facilities at the Ontario Municipal Board." In *The Place of Justice*, edited by Law Commission of Canada, 95–119. Nova Scotia: Fernwood.

– 2013. "'They Should Not be Allowed to Do This to The Homeless and Mentally Ill': Minimum Separation Distance Bylaws Reconsidered." In *Mad Matters: A Critical Reader in Canadian Mad Studies*, edited by B.A. LeFrançois, R. Menzies, G. Reaume, chapter 16. Toronto: Canadian Scholars' Press.

Finkler, L., and J. Grant. 2011. "Minimum Separation Distance Bylaws for Group Homes: The Negative Side of Planning Regulation." *Canadian Journal of Urban Research* 20, no. 1: 33–56.

Fish, V. 2004. "Some Gender Biases in Diagnosing Traumatized Women." In *Bias in Psychiatric Diagnosis*, edited by P. Caplan and L. Cosgrove, 213–20. New York: Jason Aronson

Forchuk, C., G. Nelson, and B. Hall. 2006. "'It's Important to be Proud of the Place You Live In': Housing Problems and Preferences of Psychiatric Survivors." *Perspectives in Psychiatric Care* 42, no. 1: 42–52.

Forester-Jones, R., J. Carpenter, P. Cambridge, A. Tate, A. Hallam, M. Knapp, and J. Beechham. 2002. "The Quality of Life of People 12 Years after Resettlement from Long Stay Hospitals: Users' Views on Their Living Environment, Daily Activities, and Future Aspirations." *Disability and Society* 17, no. 7: 741–58.

Forester-Jones, R., J. Carpenter, P. Coolen-Schrijner, P. Cambridge, A. Tate, A. Hallam, J. Beechham, M. Knapp, and D. Woolf. 2012. "Good Friends are Hard to Find? The Social Networks of People with Mental Illness 12 Years after Deinstitutionalization." *Journal of Mental Health* 21, no. 1: 4–14.

Foucault, M. 1970. *The Order of Things: An Archaeology of the Human Sciences*. New York: Vintage Books.

– 1977a. *Discipline and Punish*. London: Allen Lane.

– 1977b. *Language, Counter-Memory, Practice: Selected Essays and Interviews*. Oxford: Blackwell.

– 1980a. *Power/Knowledge: Selected Interviews and Other Writings 1972–1977*. Hassocks: Harvester Press.

– 1980b. *The History of Sexuality, Vol. 1*. New York: Vintage Books.

– 1984. "Space, Knowledge, and Power." In *Foucault Reader*, edited by P. Rabinow, 239–56. New York: Pantheon.

– 1987. "The Ethic of Care for the Self as a Practice of Freedom." *Philosophy and Social Criticism* 12, no. 2/3: 112–31.

– 1991a. "Governmentality." In *The Foucault Effect: Studies in Govern-mentality*, edited by G. Burchell, C. Gordon, and P. Miller, 87–104. Chicago: University of Chicago Press.

– 1991b. *The Foucault Effect*. Chicago: Chicago University Press.

– 1994. "'*Omnes et Singulatim*': Toward a Critique of Political Reason." In *Power: Essential Works of Foucault,* vol. 3, 298–325. New York: The New Press.

– 1995. *Discipline and Punish*. New York: Vintage.

– 2006. *The Hermeneutics of the Subject: Lectures at the Collège de France, 1981–82*. New York: Picador.

– 2007. *Birth of the Clinic*. London: Tavistock.

– 2008. *Psychiatric Power: Lectures at the Collège de France, 1973–74*. New York: Picador.

– 2009. *History of Madness*. London and New York: Routledge.

Freedman, J., and G. Combs. 1996. *Narrative Therapy: The Social Construction of Preferred Realities*. New York: W.W. Norton.

Freire, P. 1970. *Pedagogy of the Oppressed*. New York: The Seabury Press.

Gablick, S. 1991. *The Reenchantment of Art*. New York: Thames and Hudson.

Gall, G. 2009. *The Future of Union Organising: Building for Tomorrow*. Basingstoke: Palgrave Macmillan.

Garber O'Brien, P., and D. Tamlyn. 2010. "Nursing Practice in Canada." In *Medical-Surgical Nursing in Canada: Assessment and Management of Clinical Problems*, edited by S. Lewis, M. Heitkemper, S. Ruff Dirksen, P. Garber O'Brien, and L. Bucher, 2–18. Toronto: Elsevier.

Gardiner, M. 2004. "Wild Publics and Grotesque Symposiums: Habermas and Bakhtin on Dialogue, Everyday Life, and the Public Sphere." *The Sociological Review. Special Issue – After Habermas: New Perspectives on the Public Sphere* 52, special issue 1: 28–48.

Garland-Thomson, R. 1997. *Extraordinary Bodies: Figuring Physical Disability in American Culture and Literature*. New York: Columbia University Press.

Geddes, L. 2008. "Gene Variant More Prevalent in Transsexuals." *New Scientist* 199, no. 2667: 14.

Gibson, P.R. 2004. "Histrionic Personality Disorder." In *Bias in Psychiatric Diagnosis*, edited by P. Caplan and L. Cosgrove, 201–6. New York: Jason Aronson.

Giddens, A. 1991. *Modernity and Self-Identity: Self and Society in the Late Modern Age*. Stanford: Stanford University Press.

Ginsberg, E.K. 1996. "Introduction: The Politics of Passing." In *Passing and the Fictions of Identity*, edited by E.K. Ginsberg, 1–18. Durham and London: Duke University Press.

Glaser, B., and A. Strauss. 1968. *The Discovery of Grounded Theory*. Hawthorne: Aldine de Gruyter.

Godin, P., J. Davies, B. Heyman, L. Reynolds, A. Simpson, and M. Floyd. 2007. "Opening Communicative Space: A Habermasian Understanding of a User-led Participatory Research Project." *Forensic Psychiatry & Psychology* 18, no. 4: 452–69.

Goffman, E. 1963. *Stigma: Notes on the Management of Spoiled Identity*. Harmondsworth: Penguin. `

– 1964. *Asylums: Essays on the Social Situation of Mental Patients and Other Inmates*. New York: Anchor Books.

Gold, M. 2008. "Transportation: A Vehicle for Mental Health." *Network, Magazine of the Canadian Mental Health Association, Ontario Division* 24, no. 1: 26–7.

Goodley, D. and M. Rapley. 2001. "How Do You Understand 'Learning Difficulties'? Towards a Social Theory of Impairment." *Mental Retardation* 39, no. 3: 229–32.

Goodrum, S., D. Umberson, and K. Anderson. 2001. "The Batterer's View of the Self and Others in Domestic Violence." *Sociological Inquiry* 71, no. 2: 221–40.

Gordon, C. 1991. "Governmental Rationality: An Introduction." In *The Foucault Effect: Studies in Governmentality*, edited by G. Burchell, C. Gordon, and P. Miller, 1–48. Chicago: University of Chicago Press.

Greger, M. 1999. "Heart Failure – Diary of a Third Year Medical Student." http://www.just-think-it.com/heartfailure.pdf. Last accessed 14 October 2012.

Grobe, J., ed. 1995. *Beyond Bedlam: Contemporary Women Survivors Speak Out*. Chicago: The Third Press.

Groce, N.E. 2003 [1985]. *Everyone Here Spoke Sign Language: Hereditary Deafness on Martha's Vineyard*. Cambridge: Harvard University Press.

Habermas, J. 1976. *Legitimation Crisis*. London: Heinemann.

– 1981. "New Social Movements." *Telos* 49: 33–7.

– 1986. *The Theory of Communicative Action, vol.1: Reason and the Rationalization of Society*. Cambridge: Polity Press.

– 1987. *The Theory of Communicative Action, vol. 2: The Critique of Functionalist Reason*. Cambridge: Polity Press.

Hagen, B. 2007. "Measuring Melancholy: A Critique of the Beck Depression Inventory and Its Use in Mental Health Nursing." *International Journal of Mental Health Nursing* 16, no. 2: 105–15.

– 2008. "Let's Do Lunch?: The Ethics of Accepting Gifts from the Pharmaceutical Industry." *The Canadian Nurse* 104, no. 4: 30–5.

Haller, J.S. 1995 [1971]. *Outcasts from Evolution: Scientific Attitudes of Racial Inferiority, 1958–1900*. Urbana: University of Illinois Press.

Harley E., J. Boardman, and T. Craig. 2012. "Friendship in People with Schizophrenia." *Psychiatric Epidemiology* 47: 1291–9.

Harley, S. 1990. "For the Good of Family and Race: Gender, Work, and Domestic Roles in the Black Community, 1880–1930." *Signs* 15, no. 2: 336–49.

Hart, C. 2004. *Nurses and Alinsky Politics: The Impact of Power and Practice*. Basingstoke: Palgrave Macmillan.

Hatzfeld, J. 2005. *Machete Season: The Killers in Rwanda Speak*. New York: Picador.

Hayek, F. 2001. *The Road to Serfdom*. London: Routledge.

Healy, D. 2006. "The Latest Mania: Selling Bipolar Disorder." *PLoS Med* 3, no. 4: 23.

Heron, B. 2007. *Desire for Development: Whiteness, Gender, and the Helping Imperative*. Waterloo: Wilfred Laurier University Press.

Heslin, K.C., A.B. Hamilton, T.K. Singzon, J.L. Smith, and N.L.R. Anderson. 2011. "Alternative Families in Recovery: Fictive Kin Relationships among Residents of Sober Living Homes." *Qualitative Health Research* 21, no. 4: 477–88.

Hill Collins, P. 2000. *Black Feminist Thought: Knowledge, Consciousness, and the Politics of Empowerment*. New York: Routledge.

Hochschild, A.R. 1983. *The Managed Heart: Commercialization of Human Feeling*. Berkeley: University of California Press.

Hodge, S. 2005. "Competence, Identity, and Intersubjectivity: Applying Habermas's Theory of Communicative Action to Service User Involvement in Mental Health Policy Making." *Social Theory & Health* 3: 165–82.

– 2009. "User Involvement in the Construction of a Mental Health Charter: An Exercise in Communicative Rationality?" *Health Expectations* 12: 251–61.

Hoerr, J. 1997. "We Can't Eat Prestige: The Women Who Organized Harvard." Philadelphia: Temple University Press.

Hoffman, S. 2005. "'Racially-tailored' Medicine Unraveled." *American University Law Review* 55, no. 2: 395–452.

Hook, D. 2012. *A Critical Psychology of the Postcolonial: The Mind of Apartheid*. London and New York: Routledge.

hooks, b. 1984. *Feminist Theory: From Margin to Center*. Boston: South End Press.

Hornstein, G.A. 2009. *Agnes's Jacket: A Psychologist's Search for the Meanings of Madness*. Pennsylvania: Rodale.

Howarth, D., A. Norval, and Y. Stavrakakis, eds. 2000. *Discourse Theory and Political Analysis: Identities, Hegemonies, and Social Change.* Manchester: University of Manchester Press.

Huddart, D. 2006. *Homi K. Bhabha.* London and New York: Routledge.

– 2002. "Hunger Striker Protests Use of Physical Restraints in Group Homes." *Canadian Medical Association Journal* 167, no. 4: 386.

Ingleby, D. 2011 [1985]. "'Professionals as Socializers: The 'Psy Complex.'" In *Critical Psychology: Critical Concepts in Psychology*, edited by I. Parker, vol. 1, 279–307. London and New York: Routledge.

Inman, S. 2007. "Community Response to the 'Madness, Citizenship, and Social Justice' Conference Plans. Email Petition to Robert Menzies and Conference Sponsors and Funders." Vancouver: B C Schizophrenia Society, Vancouver/Richmond Branch, 31 October 2007.

– 2010. *After Her Brain Broke: Helping My Daughter Recover Her Sanity.* Dundas: Bridgeross Communications/Ingram Books.

Jacobson, N. 2004. *In Recovery: The Making of Mental Health Policy.* Nashville: Vanderbilt University Press.

Jarley, P. 2005. "Unions as Social Capital: Renewal through a Return to the Logic of Mutual Aid?" *Labor Studies Journal* 29, no. 4: 1–26.

Jenkins, A. 1990. *Invitations to Responsibility: The Therapeutic Engagement of Men Who Are Violent and Abusive.* Adelaide: Dulwich Centre Publications.

– 1991. "The Intervention with Violence and Abuse in Families: The Inadvertent Perpetuation of Irresponsible Behavior." *Australian and New Zealand Journal of Family Therapy* 12, no. 4: 186–95.

– 2009. *Becoming Ethical: A Parallel, Political Journey with Men Who Have Abused.* Dorset: Russell House Publishing.

Jessop, B. 2007. "From Micro-Powers to Governmentality: Foucault's Work on Statehood, State Formation, Statecraft, and State Power." *Political Geography* 26, no. 1: 34–40.

– 1901. "The Jew as a Study in Racial Pathology." *The British Medical Journal* 2, no. 2125: 828.

Jin, M. 1990. "Strangers in a Hostile Landscape." In *Creation Fire: A CAFRA Anthology of Caribbean Women's Poetry*, edited by R. Espinet, 131–2. Toronto: Sister Vision.

Johnson, B. 1987. *A World of Difference.* Baltimore: John Hopkins.

Jones, R., J. Chesters, and M. Fletcher. 2003. "Make Yourself at Home: People Living with Psychiatric Disability in Public Housing." *International Journal of Psychosocial Rehabilitation* 7: 67–79.

Jordan, B.K., W.E. Schlenger, J.A. Fairbank, and J.M. Cadell. 1996. "Prevalence of Psychiatric Disorders among Incarcerated Women." *Archives of General Psychiatry* 53, no. 6: 513–19.

Kagan, C., and M. Burton. 2000. "Prefigurative Action Research: An Alternative Basis for Critical Psychology?" *Annual Review of Critical Psychology* 2: 73–87.

Kaiser, A. 2001. "Restraint and Seclusion in Canadian Mental Health Facilities: Assessing the Prospects for Improved Access to Justice." *Windsor Yearbook of Access to Justice* 19: 391–417.

Kameny, F.E. 1965. "Civil Liberties: A Progress Report July 1965, 12." *New York Mattachine Newsletter*, 7–22.

– 2009. "How it All Started." *Journal of Gay & Lesbian Mental Health* 13, no. 2: 76–81.

Kilty, J.M. 2012. "It's Like They Don't Want You to Get Better." *Practising 'Psy' in the Carceral Context, Feminism & Psychology* 22, no. 2: 162–82.

Kirk, S., and H. Kutchins. 1992. *The Selling of DSM: The Rhetoric of Science in Psychiatry*. New Brunswick and New Jersey: Transaction Publishers.

– 1994. "The Myth of the Reliability of the DSM." *Journal of Mind and Behavior* 15: 71–86.

Kissack, T. 1995. "Freaking Fag Revolutionaries: New York's Gay Liberation Front, 1969–1971." *Radical History Review* 62, no. 62: 105–34.

Knopp, F. 1976. *Instead of Prison: A Handbook for Abolitionists*. New York: Faculty Press.

Knowles, C. 2000. *Bedlam on the Streets*. London: Routledge.

Lacan, J. 1977. *The Four Fundamental Concepts of Psycho-Analysis*, edited by Jacques-Alain Miller, translated by Alan Sheridan. London: Penguin Books.

Laclau, E., and C. Mouffe. 1985. *Hegemony and Socialist Strategy: Towards a Radical Democratic Politics*. London: Verso.

Lea, J. 1987. "Left Realism: A Defence." *Contemporary Crises* 11: 357–70.

LeFrançois, B.A. 2011. "Queering Child and Adolescent Mental Health Services: The Subversion of Heteronormativity in Practice." *Children & Society*. doi: 10.1111/j.1099-0860.2011.00371.x. Last accessed 26 April 2011.

– 2013. "Adultism." In *Encyclopedia of Critical Psychology*, edited by T. Teo. Springer Reference.

LeFrançois, B.A., R. Menzies, and G. Reaume, eds. 2013. *Mad Matters: A Critical Reader in Canadian Mad Studies*. Toronto: Canadian Scholars' Press.

Leifer, R. 1990. "Introduction: The Medical Model as the Ideology of the Therapeutic State." *Journal of Mind and Behavior* 11: 247–58.

Levine, M. 1977. "Nursing Ethics and the Ethical Nurse." *American Journal of Nursing* 77, no. 5: 845–9.

Lewis, C.S. 1970. *God in the Dock: Essays on Theology and Ethics*. Grand Rapids: Eerdmans Publishing.

Lewis, L. 2007. "Epistemic Authority and the Gender Lens." *The Sociological Review* 55, no. 2: 273–92.

Leys, C. 2003. *Market-driven Politics: Neoliberal Democracy and the Public Interest*. London: Verso.

Leys, C., and S. Player. 2011. *The Plot against the NHS*. London: Merlin Press.

Lidbetter, E.I. 1984 [1921]. "Pedigrees of Pauper Stocks." In *Eugenics, Genetics, and Family: Second International Congress of Eugenics*, New York, 22–28 September 1921, 390–3.

Loomba, A. 1998. *Colonialism/Postcolonialism*. The New Critical Idiom Series. London and New York: Routledge.

Lorde, A. 2007. *Sister Outsider: Essays and Speeches by Audre Lorde*. Berkeley: Crossing.

MacLure, M., R. Holmes, L. Jones, and C. MacRae. 2010. "Silence as Resistance to Analysis: Or, on Not Opening One's Mouth Properly." *Qualitative Inquiry* 16, no. 6: 492–500.

Mahmood, S. 2005. *The Politics of Piety: The Islamic Revival and the Feminist Subject*. Princeton: Princeton University Press.

Mandel, E. 1974. *Late Capitalism*. London: New Left Books.

– 1978. *From Stalinism to Eurocommunism: The Bitter Fruits of 'Socialism in One Country.'* London: New Left Books.

Matthews, R., and J. Young, eds. 1992. *Rethinking Criminology: The Realist Debate*. London: Sage.

McCaslin, W.D., ed. 2005. *Justice as Healing: Indigenous Ways*. St Paul: Living Justice Press.

McDonagh, P. 2008. *Idiocy: A Cultural History*. Liverpool: Liverpool University Press.

McKeown, M. 2009. "Alliances in Action: Opportunities and Threats to Solidarity between Workers and Service Users in Health and Social Care Disputes." *Social Theory & Health* 7: 148–69.

– 2012. "Linking the Academy and Activism: From Constructed Subjectivities to Participatory, Communicative Agency." PhD Thesis, University of Central Lancashire.

McKeown, M., and F. Jones, 2014. "Service User Involvement: A Critical View of Policies, Practice, and Politics." In *Mental Health Policy for Nurses*, edited by Ian Hulatt. London: Sage.

McLaughlin, T. 1996. "Coping with Hearing Voices: An Emancipatory Discourse Analytic Approach." In *Critical Psychology: Critical Concepts in Psychology*, edited by I. Parker, vol. 4, 262–9. London and New York: Routledge, 2011.

McSweeney, S. 2004. "Depression in Women." In *Bias in Psychiatric Diagnosis*, edited by P. Caplan and L. Cosgrove, 183–8. New York: Jason Aronson.

Menzies, R. 2007. "Virtual Backlash: Representations of Men's 'Rights' and Feminist 'Wrongs' in Cyberspace." In *Reaction and Resistance: Feminism, Law, and Social Change*, edited by D.E. Chunn, S.B. Boyd, and H. Lessard, 65–97. Vancouver: University of British Columbia Press.

Metzl, J.M. 2009. *The Protest Psychosis: How Schizophrenia Became a Black Disease*. Boston: Beacon.

Michener, A.J. 1998. *Becoming Anna: The Autobiography of a Sixteen Year Old*. Chicago: The University of Chicago Press.

Mifflin, E., and R. Wilton. 2005. "No Place like Home: Rooming Houses in Contemporary Urban Context." *Environment and Planning A* 37: 403–21.

Miller, J.F. 1896. "The Effects of Emancipation upon the Mental and Physical Health of the Negro of the South." *North Carolina Medical Journal* 38: 285–94.

Miller, P., and N.S. Rose. 2008. *Governing the Present: Administering Economic, Social, and Personal Life*. Cambridge: Polity.

Mills, C. 2012a. "'Special 'Treatment,' Special Rights: Dis/abled Children as Doubly Diminished Identities." In *Law and Childhood: Current Legal Issues,* vol. 14, edited by M. Freeman, 862–98. Oxford: Oxford University Press.

– 2012b. "Spoof: Faking Normal, Faking Disorder." Paper presented at Theorizing Normalcy and the Mundane: Third International Conference, "Cripping the Norm," University of Chester, UK, 26–27 June.

– 2014, forthcoming. *Decolonizing Global Mental Health: The Psychiatrization of the Majority World*. London: Routledge.

Mirowsky, J. 1990. Subjective Boundaries and Combinations in Psychiatric Diagnoses. *Journal of Mind and Behavior* 11: 407–23.

Moncrieff, J. 2003. *Is Psychiatry For Sale? An Examination of the Influence of the Pharmaceutical Industry on Academic and Practical Psychiatry*. London: Institute of Psychiatry.

Morris, J. 2011. "Rethinking Disability Policy." *Joseph Rowntree Foundation, Viewpoint:* November.

Morrison, L. J. 2003. "Talking Back to Psychiatry: Identities in the Psychiatric Consumer/Survivor/Ex Patient Movement." PhD Thesis, University of Pittsburgh.

Muir, K., K. Fisher, D. Abello, and A. Dadich. 2010. "'I Didn't Like Just Sittin' Around All Day': Facilitating Social and Community Participation Among People with Mental Illness and High Levels of Psychiatric Disability." *Journal of Social Policy* 39, no. 3: 375–91.

Nandy, A. 1983. *The Intimate Enemy: Loss and Recovery of Self under Colonialism*. Oxford: Oxford University Press.

National Council on Disability. 2006. *The Needs of People with Psychiatric Disabilities during and after Hurricanes Katrina and Rita: Position Paper and Recommendations*. Washington: National Council on Disability.

Neu, D., and R. Therrien. 2003. *Accounting for Genocide: Canada's Bureaucratic Assault on Aboriginal People*. Halifax: Fernwood.

Nussbaum, M. 2006. *Frontiers of Justice: Disability, Nationality, Species Membership*. Cambridge: The Belknap Press of Harvard University Press.

Oaks, D. 2008. "Prospects for a Nonviolent Revolution in the Mental Health System during a Time of Psychiatric Globalization." Keynote Address at the Madness, Citizenship, and Social Justice Conference, Simon Fraser University, Vancouver, 12–15 June.

Office for National Statistics. 2012. *Labour Disputes, Annual Article 2011*. London: Office for National Statistics.

Oliver, M. 1996. *Understanding Disability: From Theory to Practice*. New York: St Martin's Press.

Oliver, M., and C. Barnes. 2012. *The New Politics of Disablement*. Basingstoke: Palgrave Macmillan.

Ontario Human Rights Commission. 2012. *Minds that Matter: Report on the Consultation on Human Rights, Mental Health and Addictions*. Toronto: Ontario Human Rights Commission.

Parker, I. 2007. *Revolution in Psychology: Alienation to Emancipation*. London: Pluto Press.

Patel, S. 2009. "Encountering the Terrorism of 'Madness': The Nation's Normal Race to the Culture of Categories." Paper presented at the Society for Disability Studies Annual Conference, Tucson, 17–20 June 2009.

Paul, D. 2006. *We Were Not the Savages: Collision between European and Native American Civilizations*, 3rd edition. Halifax: Fernwood Publishing.

Penfold, P.S., and G.A. Walker. 1983. *Women and the Psychiatric Paradox*. Montreal: Open University Press.

Perlin, M. 1991. "Competency, Deinstitutionalization, and Homelessness: A Story of Marginalization." *Houston Law Review* 28: 63–142.

– 2003. "'You Have Discussed Lepers and Crooks': Sanism in Clinical Teaching." *Clinical Law Review* 9: 683–729.

Pilgrim, D. 2005. "Protest and Co-option: The Recent Fate of the Psychiatric Patient's Voice." In *Beyond the Water Towers: The Unfinished Revolution in Mental Health Services 1985–2005*, edited by A. Bell and P. Lindley, 17–26. London: Sainsbury Centre for Mental Health.

Pollock, A. 2004. *NHS plc: The Privatisation of Our Health Care*. London: Verso.

Poole, J.M., T. Jivraj, A. Arslanian, K. Bellows, S. Chiasson, H. Hakimy, J. Passini, and J. Reid. 2012. "Sanism, 'Mental Health,' and Social Work/Education: A Review and Call to Action. *Intersectionalities: A Global Journal of Social Work Analysis, Research, Polity, and Practice* 1: 20–36.

Popper, K. 1945. *The Open Society and its Enemies*. London: Routledge and Kegan Paul.

Porter, R. 2002. *Madness: A Brief History*. Oxford: Oxford University Press.

Pothier, D., and R. Devlin. 2006. "Introduction: Toward a Critical Theory of Dis-citizenship." In *Critical Disability Theory*, edited by R. Devlin and D. Pothier, 1–22. Vancouver: UBC Press.

Pranis, Kay. 2007. "Restorative Values." In *Handbook of Restorative Justice*, edited by Gerry Johnstone and Daniel W. Van Ness, 59–74. London and New York: Routledge.

Quiggin, J. 2010. *Zombie Economics: How Dead Ideas Still Walk Amongst Us*. Princeton: Princeton University Press.

Rabinor, J.R. 2004. "The 'Eating-disordered' Patient." In *Bias in Psychiatric Diagnosis*, edited by P. Caplan and L. Cosgrove, 189–92. New York: Jason Aronson.

Rabinow, P., and N. Rose, eds. 2003. *The Essential Foucault: Selections from Essential Works of Foucault, 1954–1984.* New York: The New Press.

Rahman, Q. 2005. "The Neurodevelopment of Human Sexual Orientation." *Neuroscience and Biobehavioral Reviews* 29, no. 7: 1,057–66.

Rahnema, M. and V. Bawtree, eds. 1997. *The Post-Development Reader.* London and New Jersey: Zed Books.

Raphael, D. 2007. *Poverty and Policy in Canada: Implications for Health and Quality of Life.* Toronto: Canadian Scholars' Press.

Rapley, M. 2004. *The Social Construction of Intellectual Disability.* Cambridge: Cambridge University Press.

Raskin, J.D., and A.M. Lewandowski. 2000. "The Construction of Disorder as a Human Enterprise." In *Constructions of Disorder: Meaning-making Frameworks for Psychotherapy*, edited by R.A. Neimeyer and J.D. Raskin, 15–40. Washington: American Psychological Association.

Read, J., N. Haslam, L. Sayce, and E. Davies. 2006. "Prejudice and Schizophrenia: A Review of the 'Mental Illness is an Illness like Any Other' Approach." *Acta Psychiatrica Scandinavica* 114: 303–18.

Reaume, G. 2000. *Remembrances of Patients Past: Patient Life at the Toronto Hospital for the Insane, 1870–1940.* Toronto: Oxford University Press.

– 2012. "Disability History in Canada: Present Work in the Field and Future Prospects." *Canadian Journal of Disability Studies* 1, no. 1: 35–81.

Reeve P., S. Cornell, B. D'Costa, R. Janzen, and J. Ochocka. 2002. "From Our Perspective: Consumer Researchers Speak About Their Experience in a Community Mental Health Research Project." *Psychiatric Rehabilitation Journal* 25, no. 4: 403–9.

Reicher, S. 1987. *Labour – Take the Power! An Alternative Way Forward for the Labour Party.* London: Labour Briefing.

Reville, D. 2013. "Is Mad Studies Emerging as a New Field of Inquiry?" In *Mad Matters: A Critical Reader in Canadian Mad Studies*, edited by B.A. LeFrançois, R. Menzies, and G. Reaume, chapter 12. Toronto: Canadian Scholars' Press.

Riessman, C.K. 1998. "Women and Medicalization: A New Perspective. In *Inventing Women: Science, Technology, and Gender*, edited by G. Kirkup and L.S. Keller, 123–44. Malden: Blackwell.

Rimmerman, C.A. 2008. *The Lesbian and Gay Movements: Assimilation or Liberation.* Boulder: Westview Press.

Romany, C. 1994. "State Responsibility Goes Private: A Feminist Critique of the Public/Private Distinction in International Human Rights Law." In *Human Rights of Women: National and International Perspectives*, edited by R.J. Cook, 85–115. Philadelphia: University of Pennsylvania Press.

Romme, M., S. Escher, J. Dillon, D. Corstens, and M. Morris. 2009. *Living with Voices: 50 Stories of Recovery*. Ross-on-Wye: PCCS Books.

Rose, N.S. 1996. *Inventing Ourselves: Psychology, Power, and Personhood*. Cambridge: Cambridge University Press.

– 1999a. *Governing the Soul: The Shaping of the Private Self*. London: Free Association Books.

– 1999b. *Powers of Freedom: Reframing Political Thought*. Cambridge: Cambridge University Press.

Rowbotham, S., L. Segal, and H. Wainwright. 1980. *Beyond the Fragments: Feminism and the Making of Socialism*. London: Merlin.

St-Amand, N., and E. LeBlanc. 2013. "Women in 19th Century Asylums: Three Exemplary Women; A New Brunswick Hero." In *Mad Matters: A Critical Reader in Canadian Mad Studies*, edited by B.A. LeFrançois, R. Menzies, and G. Reaume, chapter 2. Toronto: Canadian Scholars' Press.

Sartre, J.-P. 1943. *L'Être et le néant: Essai d'ontologie phénoménologique*. Paris: Gallimard.

Saussure, F. de. 1974. *Course in General Linguistics*. Glasgow: Fontana/Collins.

Sayce, L. 2000. *From Psychiatric Patient to Citizen: Overcoming Discrimination and Social Exclusion*. New York: St Martin's Press.

Schellenberg, S., and R. Barnes. 2009. *Committed to the Sane Asylum: Narratives on Mental Wellness and Healing*. Waterloo, Ontario: Wilfrid Laurier University Press.

Schneider, B. 2010. "Housing People with Mental Illnesses: The Discursive Construction of Worthiness." *Housing Theory and Society* 7, no. 4: 296–312.

Schneider, B., and C. McDonald. 2008. *Schizophrenia/Hearing [Our] Voices: Dilemmas of Care and Control*. Calgary: University of Calgary.

Schuengel C., S. Kef, S. Damen, and M. Worm. 2010. "'People Who Need People': Attachment and Professional Caregiving." *Journal of Intellectual Disability Research* 54, no. 1: 38–47.

Scott, J.C. 1990. *Domination and the Arts of Resistance: Hidden Transcripts*. Yale: Yale University Press.

Scull, A. 1977. *Decarceration: Community Treatment and the Deviant – A Radical View*. Englewood Cliff: Prentice-Hall.

Sedgwick, P. 1982. *Psychopolitics*. London: Pluto Press.

Sen, A. 2009. *The Idea of Justice*. Cambridge: The Belknap Press of Harvard University Press.

Shaikh, S.S. 2013. "Negotiating Activism: Racialized Women of Colour Navigating Relations of Ruling." PhD Thesis, Ontario Institute for Studies in Education, University of Toronto.

Sharpley, M.S., and E. Peters. 1999. "Ethnicity, Class, and Schizotypy." *Social Psychiatry and Psychiatric Epidemiology* 34: 407–12.

Shartal, S., L. Cowan, E. Khandor, and B. German. 2006. *Failing the Homeless: Barriers in the Ontario Disability Support Program for Homeless People with Disabilities*. Wellesley Institute.

Shaughnessy, P. 2001. "Not in My Back Yard: Stigma from a Personal Perspective." In *Stigma and Social Exclusion in Health Care*, edited by T. Mason, C. Carlisle, C. Watkins, and E. Whitehead, 181–9. London: Routledge.

Shaw, C., and G. Proctor. 2005. "Women at the Margins: A Critique of the Diagnosis of Borderline Personality Disorder." *Feminism & Psychology* 15: 483–9.

Shimrat, I. 1997. *Call Me Crazy: Stories From the Mad Movement*. Vancouver: Press Gang.

Shorter, E. 1997. *A History of Psychiatry: From the Era of the Asylum to the Age of Prozac*. New York: John Wiley & Sons.

Siebers, T. 2004. "Disability as Masquerade." *Literature and Medicine* 23, no. 1: 1–22.

Silverstein, C. 2008. "Are You Saying Homosexuality Is Normal?" *Journal of Gay & Lesbian Mental Health* 12, no. 3: 277–87.

Simmie, S., and J. Nunes. 2001. *The Last Taboo: A Survival Guide to Mental Health Care in Canada*. Toronto: McClellan & Stewart.

Simmons, R., M. Powell, and I. Greener, eds. 2009. *The Consumer in Public Services: Choice, Values, and Difference*. Bristol: Policy Press.

Simms, M., and J. Holgate, J. 2010. "Organising for What? Where is the Debate on the Politics of Organising?" *Work Employment & Society* 24: 157–68.

Sinson, J.C. 1993. *Group Homes and Community Integration of Developmentally Disabled People; Micro-Institutionalization?* London: Jessica Kingsley Publishers.

Smith, D.E. 1987. *The Everyday World as Problematic*. Toronto: University of Toronto Press.

– 2005. *Institutional Ethnography: A Sociology for People*. Toronto: Rowman & Littlefield.

Smith, D.E., and S.J. David. 1975. *Women Look at Psychiatry*. Vancouver: Press Gang.

Smith, G. 2006. *Erving Goffman*. London and New York: Routledge.

Sokal, A., and J. Bricmont. 1999. *Intellectual Impostures*. London: Profile Books.

Sollors, W. 1997. *Neither Black nor White yet Both: Thematic Explorations of Interracial Literature*. New York and Oxford: Oxford University Press.

Spandler, H. 2006. *Asylum to Action: Paddington Day Hospital, Therapeutic Communities, and Beyond*. London and Philadelphia: Jessica Kingsley Publishers.

– 2009. "Spaces of Psychiatric Contention: A Case Study of a Therapeutic Community." *Health & Place* 15: 672–8.

Spandler, H. and T. Calton. 2009. "Psychosis and Human Rights: Conflicts in Mental Health Policy and Practise." *Social Policy and Society* 8, no. 2: 245–56.

Steele, L., R. Glazier, and E. Lin. 2006. "Inequity in Mental Health Care under Canadian Universal Health Coverage." *Psychiatric Services* 57, no. 3: 317–24.

Strous, R.D. 2009. "To Protect or to Publish: Confidentiality and the Fate of the Mentally Ill Victims of Nazi Euthanasia." *Journal of Medical Ethics* 35: 361–4.

Sullivan, D., and L. Tifft. 2001. *Restorative Justice: Healing the Foundations of Our Everyday Lives*. Monsey: Willow Tree Press.

Survivors History Group. 2012. "Survivors History Group Takes A Critical Look at Historians." In *Critical Perspectives on User Involvement*, edited by M. Barnes and P. Cotterell, 7–18. Bristol: Policy Press.

Sweeney, A., P. Beresford, A. Faulkner, M. Nettle, and D. Rose, eds. 2009. *This Is Survivor Research*. Ross-on-Wye: PCCS Books.

Szasz, T. 1974. *The Myth of Mental Illness*. New York: Harper & Row.

– 1977a. *The Manufacture of Madness*. New York: Harper & Row.

– 1977b. *The Theology of Medicine: The Political-Philosophical of Medical Ethics*. Louisiana State University Press.

Szmukler, G. 2000. "Homicide Inquiries: What Sense Do They Make." *The Psychiatrist* no. 24: 6–10. doi: 10.1192/pb.24.1.6. Last accessed 14 March 2013.

Tam, L. 2010. "How a Counter-discourse to the Psychopathology of 'Obsessions' Departs from the Trope of 'Mad Genius': An

Autoethnographic Study of Relationality from 'Local to Universal.'"
Paper presented at Psycho UT: A Conference for Organizing Resistance
against Psychiatry, Toronto, 7–8 May 2010.

Tamboukou, M. 2003. "Genealogy/Ethnography: Finding the Rhythm."
In *Dangerous Encounters: Genealogy and Ethnography*, edited by
M. Tamboukou, and M. and S.J. Ball, 195–216. New York: Peter
Lang.

Tattersall, A. 2006. "Powerful Community Relationships and Union
Renewal in Australia." *Relations Industrielles* 61, no. 4: 589–614.

– 2010. *Power in Coalitions: Strategies for Strong Unions and Social
Change*. Sydney: Allen and Unwin.

Tazi, N. 2004. *Keywords: Truth: For a Different Kind of Globalization*,
edited by N. Tazi. New York: Other Press.

Taylor, F.J., and I. Gunn. 1999. "Homicides by People with Mental Illness:
Myth and Myth." *British Journal of Psychiatry* no. 174: 9–14.

– 1995. "Ten Things to Do Instead of Hitting." Valhalla: Sunburst Visual
Media.

Thomas, C. 2004. "Developing the Social Relational in the Social Model
of Disability: A Theoretical Agenda." In *Implementing the Social Model
of Disability: Theory and Research*, edited by C. Barnes and G. Mercer,
32–47. Leeds: Disability Press.

Thomson, S. 2011. "Out of the Fire: Women Survivors of Violence Use
Clay as a Medium for Social Change." In *Art Therapy and
Postmodernism: Creative Healing through a Prism*, edited by H. Burt,
118–34. Vancouver: Jessica Kingsley Publishers.

Titchkosky, T. 2001. "From the Field: Coming Out Disabled: The
Politics of Understanding." *Disability Studies Quarterly* 21, no. 4:
131–9.

Titchkosky, T., and R. Michalko. 2009. *Rethinking Normalcy: A Disability
Studies Reader*. Toronto: Canadian Scholars' Press.

Tutu, D. 1999. *No Future without Forgiveness*. New York: Doubleday.

Unger, R. 2004. *Handbook of the Psychology of Woman and Gender*. San
Francisco: John Wiley and Sons.

Ussher, J.M. 2011. *The Madness of Women: Myth and Experience*. New
York: Routledge.

– 1991. *Women's Madness: Misogyny or Mental Illness?* Amherst:
University of Massachusetts.

Van Daalen-Smith, C. 2011. "Waiting for Oblivion: Women's Experiences
with Electroshock." *Issues in Mental Health Nursing* 32: 457–72.

Van Daalen-Smith, C., and J. Gallagher. 2011. "Electroshock: A Discerning Review of the Nursing Literature. *Issues in Mental Health Nursing* 32, no. 4: 203–13.

Vanhala, L. 2011. *Making Rights a Reality? Disabiltiy Rights Activists and Legal Mobilization*. New York: Cambridge University Press.

Walby, S. 1993. "'Backlash' in Historical Context." In *Making Connections: Women's Studies, Women's Movements, Women's Lives*, edited by M. Kennedy, C. Lubelska and V. Walsh, 79–89. London & Washington: Taylor & Francis.

Waldram, J.B. 2004. *Revenge of the Windigo: The Construction of the Mind and Mental Health of North American Aboriginal Peoples*. Toronto: University of Toronto Press

Weeks, H., B. Heaphy, and C. Donovan. 2001. *Same Sex Intimacies: Families of Choice and Other Life Experiments*. New York: Routledge.

Weitz, D. 1997. "Electroshocking Elderly People: Another Psychiatric Abuse." *Changes: An International Journal of Psychology and Psychotherapy* 15, no. 2: 118–23.

– 2008. "Struggling against Psychiatry's Human Rights Violations: An Antipsychiatry Perspective." *Radical Psychology* 7: 7–8.

Weitz, D., M. Maddock, and L. Andre. 2010. "Strategies to Ban Electroshock." Paper presented at Psycho UT: A Conference for Organizing Resistance against Psychiatry, Toronto, 7 May.

West, W., and R. Morris, eds. 2000. *The Case for Prison Abolition*. Toronto: Canadian Scholars' Press.

White, M. 2004a. "Folk Psychology and Narrative Practice." In *Narrative Practice and Exotic Lives: Resurrecting Diversity in Everyday Life*, 59–118. Adelaide: Dulwich Centre Publications.

– 2004b. Narrative Therapy: New Modalities of Practice. Workshop at Glengarry Convention Centre, Truro, 8–9 March 2004.

– 2006. "Responding to Children Who Have Experienced Significant Trauma: A Narrative Perspective." In *Narrative Therapy with Children and their Families*, edited by M. White and A. Morgan, 85–98. Adelaide: Dulwich Centre Publications.

– 2007. *Maps of Narrative Practice*. New York: W.W. Norton.

– 2010. *Narrative Practice: Continuing the Conversation*. New York: W.W. Norton

White, M., and D. Epston. 1991. *Narrative Means to Therapeutic Ends*. New York: W.W. Norton.

Whitaker, R. 2010. *Anatomy of an Epidemic: Magic Bullets, Psychiatric Drugs, and the Astonishing Rise of Mental Illness in America*. New York: Broadway Paperbacks.

Wilchins, R. 2004. *Queer Theory, Gender Theory: An Instant Primer*. Los Angeles: Alyson Books.

Wills, J., and M. Simms. 2004. "Building Reciprocal Community Unionism in the UK." *Capital & Class* 82 (Spring): 59–84.

Withers, A. J. 2012. *Disability Politics and Theory*. Black Point: Fernwood.

Wong I.Y., J. Matejkowski, and S. Lee. 2009. "Social Integration of People with Serious Mental Illness: Network Transaction and Satisfaction." *Journal of Behavioural Health Services and Research*, 38, no. 1: 51–67.

Wood, J. 2004. "Monsters and Victims: Male Felons' Accounts of Intimate Partner Violence." *Journal of Social and Personal Relationships* 21, no. 5: 555–76.

Yeo, M., and A. Moorhouse, eds. 2002. *Concepts and Cases in Nursing Ethics*. Peterborough: Broadview Press.

Yolles, S.F. 1965. "Intervention against Poverty: A Fielder's Choice for the Psychiatrist." *American Journal of Psychiatry* 122, no. 3: 324–5.

Zaretsky, E. 1976. *Capitalism, the Family, and Personal Life*. London: Pluto Press.

Žižek, S. 2008. *Violence: Six Sideways Reflections*. London: Profile Books.

LEGAL SOURCES

Committee on the Rights of Persons with Disabilities. 2011a. *Concluding Observations on Spain*. CRPD/C/ESP/CO/1. http://www.ohchr.org/Documents/HRBodies/CRPD/6thsession/CRPD.C.ESP.CO.1_en.doc. Last accessed 12 November 2012.

– 2011b. *Concluding Observations on Tunisia*. CRPD/C/TUN/CO/1. http://www2.ohchr.org//SPdocs/CRPD/5thsession/CRPD-C-TUN-CO-1_en.doc. Last accessed 12 November 2012.

– 2012. *Concluding Observations on Peru*. CRPD/C/PER/CO/1. http://www.ohchr.org/Documents/HRBodies/CRPD/7thsession/CRPD.C.PER.CO.1-ENG.doc. Last accessed 12 November 2012.

Herczegfalvy v. Austria. Application No. 10533/83, Judgment of 24 September 1992, paras 82–3 (European Court of Human Rights). http://www.humanrights.is/the-human-rights project/humanrightscasesand materials/cases/regionalcases/europeancourtofhumanrights/nr/520. Last accessed 22 October 2012.

Municipal Act, S.O. 2001, c. 25.

Organization of American States. 1999. *Inter-American Convention on the Elimination of All Forms of Discrimination Against Persons with Disabilities*. 6 October. Guatemala City, Guatemala. http://www.ada.gov/pubs/ada.htm. Last accessed 22 October 2012.

R. v. Bell, 1979, 98 D.L.R. (3rd) 255 (Supreme Court of Canada).

Special Rapporteur on Torture and Other Cruel, Inhuman, or Degrading Treatment or Punishment. 2008. *Interim Report to the General Assembly*. A/63/175, 28 July. http://unispal.un.org/UNISPAL.NSF/0/707 AC2611E22CE6B852574BB004F4C95. Last accessed 12 November 2012.

State of New York Assembly. 2009. "An Act to Amend the Mental Hygiene Law, in Relation to the Use of Electroconvulsive Therapy," sponsored by Oritz and Robinson. http://assembly.state.ny.us/leg/?bn=A08779&term=2009. Last accessed 30 September 2012.

United Nations. 2007. *Convention on the Rights of Persons with Disabilities*. A/RES/61/106, 30 March. http://www.un.org/disabilities/convention/conventionfull.shtml. Last accessed 22 October 2012.

– 2006. *Basic Principles and Guidelines on the Right to a Remedy and Reparation for Gross Violations of International Human Rights Law and Serious Violations of International Humanitarian Law*, A/RES/60/147, 21 March. http://daccess-dds-ny.un.org/doc/UNDOC/GEN/N05/496/42/PDF/N0549642.pdf?OpenElement. Last accessed 22 October 2012.

– 1984. *Convention against Torture and Other Cruel, Inhuman, or Degrading Treatment or Punishment*, RES 39/46, 10 December. http://www2.ohchr.org/english/law/pdf/cat.pdf. Last accessed 22 October 2012.

– 1976. *International Covenant on Civil and Political Rights*, RES 2200A (XXI), 16 December. http://www2.ohchr.org/english/law/pdf/ccpr.pdf. Last accessed 22 October 2012.

United Nations High Commissioner for Human Rights. 2009. *Thematic Study by the Office of the United Nations High Commissioner for Human Rights on Enhancing Awareness and Understanding of the Convention on the Rights of Persons with Disabilities*. United Nations General Assembly, 26 January. http://www2.ohchr.org/english/bodies/hrcouncil/docs/10session/A.HRC.10.48.pdf. Last accessed 22 October 2012.

United States Department of Justice. 2009 [1990]. *Americans with Disabilities Act (ADA)*. 1 January. http://www.ada.gov/pubs/ada.htm. Last accessed 22 October 2012.

Contributors

SIMON ADAM is a nurse and nurse educator. He is currently completing his doctoral studies at the University of Toronto. Simon's research is in the area of nursing education and the teaching and learning of mental health nursing, focusing on the power relations and language in education and in clinical work. His community activism work involves working with psychiatric survivors and anti-psychiatry activists on various projects, including abolishing electroshock and restricting the psychiatric drugging of children.

ROSEMARY BARNES is a psychologist who has worked at Toronto General and Women's College Hospitals and been affiliated with the University of Toronto, York University, and the Ontario Institute for Studies in Education. She is currently in independent practice. She is co-author of *Committed to the Sane Asylum: Narratives on Mental Wellness and Healing.*

PETER BERESFORD OBE is professor of social policy and director of the Centre for Citizen Participation at Brunel University. He is also a long-term user of mental health services and chair of Shaping Our Lives, the UK independent disabled people's and service users' organization and network. He has a longstanding involvement in issues of participation as a service user, educator, researcher, writer, and activist. He is author of *A Straight Talking Guide to Being a Mental Health Service User* (PCCS Books, 2010).

BONNIE BURSTOW is a long-time faculty member in the Department of Leadership, Higher and Adult Education, in the Ontario

Institute for Studies in Education at the University of Toronto. A prolific scholar, her most well-known work is *Radical Feminist Therapy: Working in the Context of Violence* (Sage, 1992), and her most recent work is "A Rose by Any Other Name: Naming and the War against Psychiatry" in *Mad Matters* (2013). She has chaired many organizations involved in antipsychiatry organizing, including Coalition against Psychiatric Assault, Resistance against Psychiatry, and Ontario Coalition against Electroshock.

PAULA J. CAPLAN, PhD, is a clinical and research psychologist, advocate and activist, and Associate at Harvard University's DuBois Institute.

CHRIS CHAPMAN is assistant professor of social work at York University and holds a PhD in sociology and equity studies from OISE/UT. His research explores how ethical self-governance and interlocking oppression interact with one another. Examples of his publications are: *Colonialism, Disability, and Possible Lives* (2012) and *Fostering a Personal-is-Political Ethics: Reflexive Conversations in Social Work Education* (2013; with Nazia Hoque and Louise Utting). He is co-editor of *Disability Incarcerated: Imprisonment and Disability in the United States and Canada* (2014, Palgrave Macmillan; with Liat Ben-Moshe and Allison C. Carey).

MARK CRESSWELL is a sociologist at Durham University, UK. He is the author of many papers on the history and politics of psychiatry, the representation of trauma in the cinema, and the theory and practice of critical pedagogy.

SHAINDL DIAMOND is a psychologist practicing in Toronto, Canada. She has worked as an activist in the psychiatric survivor/mad/antipsychiatry community over the past decade. Shaindl has co-organized numerous community events including a global conference about resistance against psychiatric oppression and a feminist global campaign against ECT.

CHAVA FINKLER is an independent researcher and former Trudeau Scholar. She has published widely in areas pertaining to disability, human rights, and more recently, about land use law and affordable housing. Her article in Plan Canada entitled "Planning vs

Human Rights" (about discriminatory zoning affecting psychiatric survivors) won a best article award from the Canadian Institute of Planners in 2013.

AMBROSE KIRBY is a community activist, educator, and psychotherapist in private practice. Co-empowerment, self-determination, shamelessness, integration, interdependence, and freedom are themes he addresses in his work. He is studying at the Gestalt Institute of Toronto and has a Masters of Education in Counselling Psychology from the University of Toronto.

BRENDA A. LeFRANÇOIS is a faculty member in the School of Social Work at Memorial University of Newfoundland. She is an activist who has contributed to organizing against psychiatry on two different continents. She is co-editor (with Robert Menzies and Geoffery Reaume) of the recently released book *Mad Matters: A Critical Reader in Canadian Mad Studies*, and is guest editor (with Vicki Coppock) of the 2014 special issue of *Children and Society* on the topic of "Psychiatrised Children and their Rights: Global Perspectives."

ROBERT MENZIES is professor of sociology at Simon Fraser University. Over the past three decades he has written extensively on the history of madness and legal order, the relationship between mental health and criminal justice systems, and the sociology of academic criminology. He is the author or editor of nine books including, most recently, *Mad Matters: A Critical Reader in Canadian Mad Studies* (co-edited with Brenda A. LeFrançois, Robert Menzies, Geoffrey Reaume, Canadian Scholars' Press, 2013). Among other projects, he is currently preparing a book on the cultural and institutional history of "criminal insanity" in British Columbia.

MICK MCKEOWN has been a union activist for all of his working life, about thirty years, joining on his first day in work and becoming a steward shortly after. His current job is principal lecturer, School of Health, University of Central Lancashire, Preston, UK. He has published widely and co-ordinated the production of the collectively written text: *Service User and Career Involvement in Education for Health and Social Care* (Wiley-Blackwell). Mick is very interested in making links between trade unions and communities and has visited Canada to meet with community activists from the mental health survivor movement.

KATE MILLETT, one of the most well-known radical feminists as well as one of the most respected psychiatric survivors in the world, was part of the historical Foucault Tribunal. A prolific author, she is famous for ground-breaking books such as *Sexual Politics* (Urbana: University of Illinois Press, 2000).

CHINA MILLS is a researcher working on social isolation, shame, and humiliation as "missing dimensions" of poverty analysis, at Oxford Poverty and Human Development Initiative (OPHI). China has just completed her first book, *Decolonizing Global Mental Health: The Psychiatrization of the Majority World*, published by Routledge. Her research interests span interdisciplinary approaches to exploring the interconnections and entanglements between Global Mental Health, psychiatry, the pharmaceutical industry, and colonialism.

TINA MINKOWITZ is a human rights lawyer and was one of the drafters of the Convention on the Rights of Persons with Disabilities. She is President of the Center for the Human Rights of Users and Survivors of Psychiatry and International Representative of the World Network of Users and Survivors of Psychiatry. She continues to work for full compliance with standards set by the CRPD on the global level and in the United States. See www.chrusp. org, http://wgwnusp2013.wordpress.com and http://www. madinamerica.com/author/tminkowitz/.

IAN PARKER is Professor of Management at the University of Leicester. He is a practising psychoanalyst in Manchester. His most recent book was *Lacanian Psychoanalysis: Revolutions in Subjectivity* (Routledge, 2011).

SUSAN SCHELLENBERG is an artist and writer who began her career as a public nurse. She co-authored *Committed to the Sane Asylum: Narratives on Mental Wellness and Healing*. Her Shedding Skins dream art and text is on permanent exhibit at the Centre for Addiction and Mental Health, Clarke site, in Toronto and can be viewed online at www.susanschellenberg.com.

HELEN SPANDLER is a reader in mental health in the School of Social Work at the University of Central Lancashire, Preston, England. She has written extensively about alternative and innovative approaches to mental health care. She is currently editing a new book about the links between distress, madness, and disability (Policy Press, forthcoming). Helen is also involved in the UK-based *Asylum: The Magazine for Democratic Psychiatry* www.asylumonline.net hspandler@uclan.ac.uk

A.J. WITHERS is a queer, trans, and disabled anti-poverty and disability justice community organizer. They are the author of *Disability Politics and Theory* and the *If I Can't Dance, Is It Still My Revolution?* blog (http://still.my.revolution.tao.ca/). They are currently a PhD student at York University.

Index

96–113; public, 96; research
into, 97, 102, 108, 112n1; supportive, 96, 108 (*see also* boarding homes; group homes;
nursing homes); for youth, 99.
See also homelessness, rights

Icarus Project, 25
Ideology and Consciousness, 55
impairment, 86, 99, 112n3, 116,
117, 118, 130, 131; cognitive,
117; intellectual, 117; mobility,
102, 103, 107; perceived, 86; of
self-image, 123; as socially constructed, 116, 120
incarceration, penal, 17, 26; psychiatric, 3, 12, 26, 70, 129;
racialized, 134. *See also* committal; confinement; detention; hospitalization, institutionalization;
prison
independence, personal, 107–8,
139, 153; institutional 139,
141
Indigenous people, 12, 13, 222. *See
also* Aboriginal Canadians
inequality, 26, 198, 201, 205, 218,
221; structural, 196, 197, 213.
See also equality
injustice, 17, 131, 134, 200, 203.
See also justice
insanity, 19, 134, 195, 211, 212,
213, 214, 221, 223n4, 224n8.
See also madness; sanity
institutionalization, 4, 23, 42,
136, 195, 197, 201. *See also*
committal; confinement; deinstitutionalization; detention;
hospitalization; incarceration;
institutions

institutions, 71, 72, 73, 92, 99,
103, 196; acute care, 69, 70,
76n4; educational, 53, 56, 84,
89, 92; group homes as, 99, 102,
106, 109, 110; health care, 66,
73, 75, 145; residential care,
103; psychiatric, 20, 37, 40, 67,
121, 169, 171, 175n3, 208; public, 156, 188; ruling, 194; societal, 201; total, 20; welfare, 145.
See also deinstitutionalization;
hospitals; institutionalization
Intentional Peer Support, 134, 135
International Network toward
Alternatives and Recovery, 87
interventions, 198, 219; colonialist,
33n3, 213; crisis, 28; critical,
114; early, 81; forced, 133, 136,
137–8, 140, 143–4n18; invasive,
83; nursing, 70, 72, 74; professional, 30; psychiatric, 28, 117,
194–9, 201, 205n1; state, 78.
See also treatment
irrationality, 15n1, 95n14, 160,
196, 214, 219. See also
rationality.
isolation, 92, 108, 134, 136 164,
182; of children, 12, 15n2; of
elders, 15n2. *See also* alienation

Jarley, Paul, 154
Jenkins, Alan, 21, 25
justice, 22, 26, 66, 71, 87, 134,
140, 143n13, 155, 175, 200,
203; restorative, 134, 135, 139,
142n9; social, 57, 61, 82, 88, 93,
111. *See also* injustice; Madness,
Citizenship, and Social Justice
conference; Psychologists for
Social Justice and Equality

nursing homes, 110, 196
Nussbaum, Martha, 132

Oaks, David, 43, 88, 92
objectification, 19, 20, 82, 85, 131, 138, 215
On Our Own, 107
oppression, 5, 14, 20, 31, 33n3, 34, 46, 47, 51n5, 51n10, 62, 63, 78, 83, 88, 93, 97, 112n2, 116–20, 125, 198–203, 205, 207, 215, 217, 223; children and, 11, 33n3; colonial, 210; diagnostic, 47, 51n8, 170; disability and, 114–27; institutional, 139; internalized, 106; medicalization of, 48, 194, 203; normalization of, 18, 27; patriarchal, 197, 198; psychiatric, 3, 4, 13, 46, 47, 51n6, 82, 91, 122, 129–41, 155, 195, 199, 200, 203–4, 215; psychiatrized people and, 115; psychic, 216; systemic, 25, 27, 28, 33n3, 46, 47, 87, 139, 200, 203; LGBTQ people and, 47, 48, 168, 170, 172, 173, 194; of women, 47, 51n8, 195–9, 202. *See also* pathologization; solidarity

Packard, Elizabeth, 4
Paddington Day Hospital, 148–9
partnerships. *See* psychiatric survivor alliances
passing, gender and, 173; psychiatric drugs and, 223; as normal, 194, 210–12, 220 (*see also* normalcy); as white, 210, 211, 212 (*see also* racism)
passivity, 77, 150, 155, 156, 217, 219

paternalism, 11, 139. *See also* patriarchy
pathologization, 4, 7, 25, 26, 57–8, 76, 119, 123, 163, 169, 195, 201–5, 219; of children, 25, 30, 33n3; of disability, 119, 121, 123; of oppressed groups, 47, 121, 198, 203; of poverty, 204; psychiatric, 123, 169, 202; of racialized people, 204, 221; of resistance, 63, 83, 172; of LGBTQ people, 51n8, 122–4, 128nn12–13, 163, 165, 170–3, 206–7n8; of women, 195, 200, 204, 205. *See also* disability; medicalization; psychiatrization; psychologization
patriarchy, 4, 7, 14, 109, 110, 194, 196, 197, 202. See also oppression; paternalism; violence
Pengilly, Mary Huestis, 4
Perlin, Michael, 5, 102
pharmaceutical industry, 11, 14, 43, 66, 69, 81, 82, 94n5, 187, 218, 222. *See also* funding; psychiatric drugs
pharmacology, 5, 68, 69, 71, 72, 73, 209, 219
Phoenix Rising: The Voice of the Psychiatrized, 36
pills, hiding, 209, 214, 223
police, psychiatric role of 71, 73
politicization, 6, 85, 151, 161. *See also* depoliticization; disability
Pollock, Alyson, 151
Poole, Jennifer, 6
Popper, Karl, 158
Porter, Helen, 190
Porter, Roy, 3

service consumers. *See* consumers

service providers, 85, 98, 107; advocacy by, 107; dependency on, 98, 109, 148, 155, 165; feminist, 201–2, 205. *See also* counsellors; nurses; professionals; psychologists; social workers; workers

Service User Research Enterprise (SURE) project, 88

service users, 4, 6, 53, 61, 77–9, 80, 85–95, 108, 129, 147, 152, 153, 155, 159–60. *See also* consumers; c/s/x/m people; mad people; psychiatric survivors; psychiatrized people; social movements; user/survivors

sexism, 5, 7, 97, 107, 112n2, 115, 128n17, 194, 197, 204, 207; psychiatric, 48. *See also* discrimination; heterosexism

sexuality, 123, 176n10, 196; denial of, 109, 110

sex work. *See* workers

sheltered workshops, 97

Sherbourne Health Centre, 163, 170, 175n2, 176n9. *See also* treatment centres

Shimrat, Irit, 5

Shorter, Edward, 3

Silverstein, Charles, 123–4, 128n16

slavery, 210

Smith, Dorothy, 5, 67, 68, 69, 73, 76n3, 87

Smith, Helen, 109

social assistance, 98, 126, 148, 164, 175n4, 196. *See also* welfare

social care, 77, 151, 152, 156. *See also* social work

social change, 87, 93, 115, 146, 174, 204, 205

social control, 33n3, 98, 102, 109. *See also* psychiatry

social movements, 5–12, 35, 36, 87, 92, 93, 114, 131, 132, 146, 147, 149, 152, 155–6, 200; anti-pathologization, 122; antipsychiatry, 8, 11, 34–5, 38–9, 67, 81, 87, 118, 182, 195; anti-capitalist, 152; children and, 15n2; children's rights, 12; consumer, 114; c/s/x/m, 115–18, 120–1, 125, 126; disability rights, 8, 79, 93, 115, 125, 132, 135, 152, 156, 160, 162n6; ex-patient, 114, 206n8; feminist, 8, 199, 202; gay liberation, 8; gay rights, 122–5, 128n17, 203, 206–7n8; global democracy, 92; labour, 7–8, 145, 147, 152, 156, 158; LGBTQ emancipation; mad, 8, 31, 37, 40, 50; Mad Pride, 50; 114; Occupy, 141, 146; penal reform, 135; post-colonialism, 93; prison-abolition, 38, 135; psychiatric survivor, 5, 8, 10, 50, 81, 85, 114, 125, 126, 141, 145, 147, 149, 150, 153, 155–8, 160, 182, 192; radical, 115; restorative justice, 135; service user, 78, 79; trans, 8; user/survivor, 59, 79

socialism, 5, 62. *See also* Marxism

social work, education in, 9, 17, 31, 33n7, 90; with children, 11; psychiatric, 52. *See also* social care; social workers

social workers, 31, 78, 147, 179, dissident, 67; radical, 75, 179;

Women's Counselling, Referral,
and Education Centre (WCREC),
202
workers, knowledge, 84; mental
health, 9, 17, 22–32, 136, 145–
61 (*see also* psychiatric survivor
alliances); sex, 124, 164, 207;
welfare, 104. *See also* counsellors; nurses; professionals; psychiatric survivor alliances;
service providers; social workers

World Network of Users and
Survivors of Psychiatry, 87,
137, 141

Young, Iris, 162n9
Young, Sherri, 33
Youth in Care Canada, 205

Zucker, Ken, 169, 170